NewHope
FOR PEOPLE WITH
Diabetes

Porter Shimer

Foreword and Medical Review by
Gerald Bernstein, M.D.

PRIMA PUBLISHING

My sincere thanks to my wife, Claire, for her technical and emotional support, and to my infant son and part-time office mate, Michael, for making sure my mouse cord was always firmly attached

PRIMA PUBLISHING and colophon are trademarks of Random House, Inc., registered with the United States Patent and Trademark Office.

Published by Prima Publishing, Roseville, California. Member of the Crown Publishing Group, a division of Random House, Inc.

All products mentioned in this book are trademarks of their respective companies. This book is an independent publication and is not affiliated with or sponsored by such companies.

In order to protect their privacy, the names of some individuals cited in this book have been changed.

Interior design by Peri Poloni, Knockout Design
Illustrations by Laurie Baker-McNeile

Information about the use of herbs and nutritional supplements in chapter 7 is courtesy of *The Natural Pharmacist: Complementary Treatments for Diabetes, Revised 2nd Edition* (Roseville, CA: Prima, 1999).

Warning—Disclaimer
This book is not intended to provide medical advice and is sold with the understanding that the publisher and the author are not liable for the misconception or misuse of information provided. The author and Random House shall have neither liability nor responsibility to any person or entity with respect to any loss, damage, or injury caused or alleged to be caused directly or indirectly by the information contained in this book or the use of any products mentioned. Readers should not use any of the products discussed in this book without the advice of a medical professional.

Library of Congress Cataloging-in-Publication Data
Shimer, Porter.
    New hope for people with diabetes : your friendly authoritative guide to the latest in traditional and complementary solutions / Porter Shimer.
        p.   cm. — (New hope series)
    Includes bibliographical references and index.
    ISBN 0-7615-2571-8
    1. Diabetes—Popular works. I. Title. II. Series.
RC660.4 .S554 2001
616.4'62—dc21   2001021482

01 02 03 04 DD 10 9 8 7 6 5 4 3 2 1
Printed in the United States of America

Visit us online at www.primapublishing.com

Contents

Foreword

PLAGUE, POLIO, CHOLERA, influenza, and even mad cow disease: These are all plagues that drew headlines over the centuries and had people frightened and agitated.

We are now faced with an epidemic that is beyond the scope of all of these others—the epidemic of diabetes mellitus. Some 18 million people in the United States likely have diabetes, 95 percent being type 2. Recent data show that the number of people with this disease increased by over 6 percent per year the last 2 years. Even a conservative estimate places the number of people with diabetes in 25 years at 50 million, at a cost of $1 trillion, up from the $100 billion of 2001.

What has accounted for this increase? We are hunter-gatherers by nature, and our bodies have evolved to survive the conditions of the world hundreds of thousands of years ago. At that time, food was difficult to come by, requiring a great deal of physical labor to obtain. Therefore, many of the elements that contribute to bringing out type 2 diabetes were not present—that is, obesity, sedentary behavior, and old age. It is likely that a mutation resulted in some people being able to function a little better and survive longer. This mutation has been called the "thrifty gene." Very simply, people who burned fat more efficiently got more energy for the same amount of calories, allowing them to go without food a few extra days before a new food supply was found. This valuable asset then multiplied in the population, and it is prevalent today.

The problem is that most of us no longer have to forage for our food or fight an animal to get meat. A simple car or bus ride to the market makes everything available with little physical effort. Machines have significantly reduced needs for physical labor. As a result, most of us eat more calories than we burn, resulting in the deposition of fat. Excess weight, in turn, creates resistance to insulin and a rise in blood glucose.

Nothing is wrong with sugar, but an elevated level in the blood acts as a poison, both acutely and especially chronically. Diabetes is still the leading cause of new cases of blindness, kidney failure, and nontraumatic limb loss in the United States and a major cause of heart disease. A visit to any coronary care unit or a cardiac surgery recovery room will reveal that, on average, about 60 percent of the patients there have diabetes. Fortunately, we have many forms of treatment other than behavior changes, insulin, and many different pills. Two critically important components of treatment for people with diabetes are self-testing and education. Informed patients have a better likelihood of truly taking control of their situations.

In this book, Porter Shimer takes you through the story of diabetes. You will find history, physiology, treatments, and all the essential material you need to be master of your own fate. The complications of diabetes are preventable if blood glucose is controlled. Reading this book will help you achieve this goal.

> —Gerald Bernstein, M.D., F.A.C.P.,
> past president, American Diabetes Association,
> associate clinical professor, Albert Einstein
> College of Medicine, senior endocrinologist,
> Beth Israel Medical Center, New York

Acknowledgments

This book would not have been possible without the help of Dr. Gerald Bernstein, Susan Silva, Jamie Miller, Marjorie Lery, Alice Feinstein, Mark Hurlbert, Bob Hanisch, Dr. Warren Scott, Linda McClure, Dr. Anne Peters, Carol Bush, Jackie Owens, Pat Henshaw, Dave Kvitne, Liz Daily, Dr. Corina Graziani, Diane Quagliani, Dr. Francine Kaufman and Guy Hornsby. My sincere thanks to all.

Introduction

As a health journalist for the past 23 years, I've written about every major disease. But never one like diabetes. Never one that can be so monstrous—or so manageable. And never one that puts the responsibility for this management so firmly in the hands of the patient. With most other diseases, treatment is the duty of our doctors. With diabetes, however, treatment is our job, and while this role can feel like a tremendous burden sometimes, we need to remember how lucky we are to have this ability at all. As recently as 80 years ago, diabetes was a death sentence, but now it's merely an inconvenience requiring just a few minutes of self-care a day. Can you imagine how much someone with cancer, or multiple sclerosis, or Parkinson's disease, or AIDS would like to be able to say that about the conditions that threaten them?

As you'll learn in the pages ahead, the ability we now have to control diabetes has been one of modern medicine's great victories, but it's a victory that can't be won without you. Yes, your life will need to be different because you have diabetes, but that doesn't mean it has to be worse. It can be decidedly better, in fact, because many of the changes you'll be encouraged to make are changes we should *all* be making to lead healthier lives. Eating a nutritious low-fat diet, getting regular exercise, maintaining a healthy weight, and learning to deal effectively with stress are the staples of health and longevity for all of us, not just those who have lost the ability to metabolize glucose.

Diabetes now can be managed so effectively, in fact, that people who control their conditions well can expect to live longer than their non-diabetic peers who take their health for granted by smoking, drinking too much, or being overweight. And if you're currently leading such a lifestyle yourself, you might want to think of your diabetes as a blessing in disguise for the incentive it can give you to change your ways.

If this is beginning to sound like an overly optimistic spin to put on such a depressingly debilitating disease, it isn't—and plenty of real-life examples prove it. There's not a walk of life, in fact, in which people with diabetes haven't made great strides: Thomas Edison, Ty Cobb, Ernest Hemingway, Jackie Robinson, Paul Cézanne, H. G. Wells, James Cagney, Arthur Ashe, Billie Jean King, Elizabeth Taylor, Ella Fitzgerald, Jackie Gleason, Dizzie Gillespie, Jack Benny, Elvis Presley, Johnny Cash, Halle Barry, Mary Tyler Moore, and Olympic gold medal swimmer Gary Hall. Do these sound like sick people to you?

If so, then maybe we should all be so ill. These people went on to do great things despite their diabetes, and maybe even because of it. Who's to say, after all, that the success these people achieved in their careers wasn't due in part to the same diligence they employed to succeed against their disease? "Adversity doth best discover virtue," as Francis Bacon observed, and with diabetes this adage is most definitely true. The disease has a way of giving a crash course in some of life's most important lessons—things like the value of working hard, maintaining a positive attitude, accepting support from others, and taking time to smell those proverbial roses. Yes, your diabetes is going to ask you to face challenges, but with those challenges will come opportunities for victories you might not otherwise have been inspired to win.

What it takes to succeed against diabetes, in other words, is what it takes to succeed in life. To whatever degree this book might help in either of those quests would give me a satisfaction I haven't the words to express.

CHAPTER 1

Diabetes 101

✑

THAT DIABETES WILL directly or indirectly take the lives of an estimated 200,000 Americans this year attests to its power to deceive. Diabetes deceives us into feeling we're healthy when we're not. It deceives us into thinking it's not a serious problem when it is. It deceives us into thinking we can't make a difference in its outcome when we most definitely can. Much of the hope that exists for overcoming diabetes, in fact, depends on our willingness to accept responsibility for the disease. We don't "catch" diabetes, you see, nor do we necessarily inherit it. Genes may establish a predisposition for the disease, but by far the most common form of diabetes—known as type 2—is a condition we, for the most part, bring on ourselves.

If that sounds like a bitter pill to swallow, it shouldn't, because it means no one is in a better position to control diabetes than we are. If there's a disease that grants power to the patient, it's diabetes. Our doctors can coach us in managing the illness and provide us with the appropriate medications, but the day-to-day battles against diabetes must be fought, and won, by us. As Richard S. Beaser, M.D., chair of the Patient Education Committee at the Joslin Diabetes Center in Boston, says, what we do for ourselves in learning to manage diabetes isn't just part of the treatment—it *is* the treatment.

So get ready to learn. In this chapter we'll look at just how serious a problem diabetes has become, who's getting the disease and why. We'll also examine the differences between the two primary types of diabetes (type 1 and type 2), looking at their most common symptoms and the complications they can cause. We'll even learn a little about the history of diabetes, described as a disease that causes the body to "melt" away by the ancient Egyptians as long ago as 1550 B.C.

Before reading as much as another word, however, keep in mind that millions of people throughout the United States and the world have diabetes yet are living healthy, happy, and productive lives. It's all about effort and attitude. If there's a will, there are countless ways our war against diabetes can be won.

A GROWING BUT PREVENTABLE PROBLEM

For a disease that, according to a recent survey by the American Diabetes Association (ADA), is considered a "serious" health problem by only 13 percent of the U.S. population, diabetes is causing a lot of serious ill health. Heart attacks, strokes, blindness, limb amputations, kidney failure, digestive disorders, gum disease, bladder infections, urinary incontinence, carpal tunnel syndrome, fatigue, irritability, and sexual dysfunction in men and women alike—diabetes can directly or indirectly cause these problems, and more. According to some estimates, diabetes currently is the third leading cause of death by disease in the United States, behind only heart disease and cancer. Most worrisome of all, the disease appears to be on a dramatic rise.

As many as five million people may have diabetes without knowing it.

The number of people with diabetes in the United States has tripled since 1960. Currently about 800,000 new cases are diagnosed every year, with the number of known cases as of the spring of 2001 estimated at about 11 million. That figure doesn't tell the whole story, however, given that as many as five million people may have diabetes without knowing it. These are the cases that have medical authorities most concerned, because diabetes can do considerable damage before causing symptoms noticeable enough to alert people to seek treatment.

"Of course it's tragic," says Corina Graziani, M.D., who sees the devastation of this disease every day as a diabetes educator and clinical assistant professor of family medicine at Thomas Jefferson University Hospital in Philadelphia. "So much of the disability and hardship that diabetes causes could be prevented if more people would get themselves diagnosed and begin treatment in time."

Also tragic—and largely preventable—is how type 2 diabetes in recent years has begun to inch its way down the age ladder. Once a problem mostly for people 45 and older, type 2 diabetes is now occurring with alarming frequency in people as young as their teens. The illness is becoming "a disease of the young," remarked the dean of the Mount Sinai School of Medicine, Arthur Rubenstein, M.D., to *Newsweek* magazine in the fall of 2000, when the Centers for Disease Control and Prevention (CDC) released news of the changing demographics of this once-designated "adult-onset" disease.

> *So much of the disability and hardship that diabetes causes could be prevented if more people would get themselves diagnosed and begin treatment in time.*
>
> —CORINA GRAZIANI, M.D.

No longer. In light of the recent migration of type 2 diabetes into younger groups, the American Diabetes Association in 1999 chose to drop the "adult-onset" tag to prevent giving a false impression of who's at risk. The disease now seems to be striking old and young alike, as shown by the CDC's surprising and worrisome findings. While the CDC found that diabetes increased within the general population by 33 percent between 1990 and 1998, for example, they found an increase over twice that great—70 percent—in people ages 30 to 39, a group formerly considered relatively immune (see figure 1.1). Mincing no words, the CDC's diabetes director, Frank Vinicor, M.D., called the increase an "explosion."

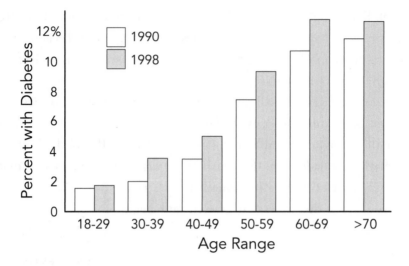

Figure 1.1—*Prevalence of Diabetes by Age*

Source: Centers for Disease Control and Prevention

"DIABESITY" AND "SYNDROME X"

Why should this disease be suddenly claiming younger victims?

For the answer to this important question, the latest research suggests we may need to look no further than our waistlines. Type 2 diabetes—by far the most common type and hence the primary focus of this book—has been increasing largely because our body weights have been increasing, and not just in those of us old enough to retire to our easy chairs. Studies show that being overweight increases risks for type 2 diabetes more than any other factor within our power to control, and more and more younger Americans, unfortunately, are falling prey.

A recent study by the CDC reported in the *Journal of the American Medical Association*, for example, found that while rates of obesity among the general population have risen by almost 50 percent since 1990, the greatest increases have been in people between the ages of

18 and 29. "Obesity can increase risks for type 2 diabetes at any age, and the new statistics are proving it," says Gerald Bernstein, M.D., former president of the American Diabetes Association, now a senior endocrinologist at the Beth Israel Medical Center in New York.

Obesity can begin to sow the seeds for diabetes so early, in fact, that even in children who are obese, research shows that fully 60 percent will have a risk factor for diabetes by the age of 10. Should it come as any surprise, then, that in adults with diabetes, an estimated 90 percent will be at least 20 percent overweight? Yes, obesity can have genetic roots in some cases, Dr. Bernstein says, but mostly it's our high-calorie, low-activity lifestyles that are to blame. "We're simply eating too much and exercising too little, and it's upsetting some of the most basic biochemical mechanisms responsible for keeping us alive."

Especially risky for the development of type 2 diabetes, studies show, is what's known as *visceral* or *truncal obesity*, in which excess fat is carried mainly in the area of the abdomen as opposed to lower down, in the area of the hips or thighs. Because this type of obesity puts more fat in the immediate area of the liver, the fat has a greater tendency to find its way into the liver's blood supply, thus interfering with sensitive hormonal processes required for proper glucose regulation. Studies show, too, that people who gain weight later in life—such as when we adopt our lounge-chair lifestyles—are more apt to accumulate the weight in the area of the abdomen, and hence increase risks for diabetes, than people who have been overweight since childhood.

> *Being overweight increases risks for type 2 diabetes more than any other factor within our power to control.*

The link between diabetes and abdominal obesity brought on by the quintessential "couch potato" lifestyle is now so well established, in fact, that the term *diabesity* has been coined. "These people frequently will have high blood pressure and high blood fats, as well,"

Dr. Bernstein says, "thus constituting a very risky situation, referred to as *syndrome X*, which increases the risk of developing heart disease.

NO ORGAN UNTOUCHED

Obesity and inactivity aren't the only factors associated with type 2 diabetes, of course, but they can be the final straws that bring the disease on, says Francine Kaufman, M.D., director of the Comprehensive Childhood Diabetes Center, professor of pediatrics, and head of the endocrinology department at the University of Southern California School of Medicine. "Diabetes is an incredibly complex disease that we still don't fully understand, but we do know that it's far more prevalent in industrialized countries where high standards of living tend to make overeating and sedentary lifestyles more common," she notes.

The link between diabetes and abdominal obesity brought on by the quintessential "couch potato" lifestyle is now so well established, in fact, that the term diabesity *has been coined.*

Too much of "the good life" for our own good, in other words, and with some potentially very heavy dues to pay. For a disease that can be so effortless to contract, diabetes can take an exhausting toll, leading to a dizzying array of complications if permitted to run its course. For a list of the most common consequences of diabetes, and how likely they are to occur, check the sidebar "Harmful from Head to Toe." Keep in mind as you do, however, that the risks for developing every one of these complications, as proven by research we'll be looking at shortly, can be greatly reduced or even eliminated entirely if diabetes is diagnosed and treated before becoming firmly entrenched.

FINICKY CELLS, "STICKY" BLOOD

So what could possibly go wrong to wreak such full-body havoc?

In someone with diabetes, the body's cells essentially lose their "appetites." Normally the body's cells are gluttons for glucose, also called *blood sugar,* which is released into the bloodstream following digestion of the food we eat. But in the diabetic body, cells pass glucose by. Not only does this leave cells short on energy, thus compromising the functioning of some of the body's most vital systems, it leaves the unconsumed glucose in the bloodstream waiting. And waiting.

This is when trouble begins. As helpful as glucose can be when it's being accepted by the body's cells, it can be very disruptive indeed when it's not. Glucose is a modified form of sugar, after all, so when levels in the blood get too high (above approximately 126 milliliters of glucose per deciliter of blood for extended periods), blood cells can begin to become "sticky" and cease to circulate as freely as they should. The result of this impaired circulation—and especially when compounded by dehydration, which is not uncommon with diabetes—is that certain tissue can become seriously deprived of vital nutrients and oxygen, causing what's known as *necrosis,* a condition that can require affected extremities to be amputated in severe cases.

Glucose-laden blood also can impart its stickiness to molecules of protein that help make up the body's various types of tissue, thus adding an additional level of havoc as these molecules can begin to bind to others, creating circulatory logjams that can impair the function of such vital organs as the kidneys and liver. Particles of fat in the blood also can become sticky, and hence more likely to attach to blood vessel walls, increasing risks of heart attacks and strokes as the blood vessels can

> *When glucose levels in the blood get too high, blood cells can begin to become "sticky" and cease to circulate as freely as they should.*

narrow and eventually clog. As we'll be seeing in more detail in chapter 5, this is why people with type 2 diabetes are advised to reduce the fat in their diets—to give glucose less to hang on artery walls.

But why should cells be reluctant to "eat" their glucose in the first place? Cells might be considered finicky in the sense that they will refuse to consume glucose unless the glucose is accompanied by a hormone produced by the pancreas called *insulin.* Insulin's job is to

Harmful from Head to Toe

For the estimated 87 percent of the population not convinced that diabetes can be a serious medical problem, the following list should be instructive. Left to run its ruinous course, diabetes can mount an attack quite literally from head to toe.

Brain. Diabetes can increase risk of stroke by as much as fivefold, and new research suggests it may increase risks for Alzheimer's disease as well.

Eyes. Diabetes is the leading cause of blindness in people between the ages of 20 and 74, causing as many as 24,000 new cases every year.

Mouth. Diabetes increases risk of gum disease by reducing the body's ability to fight infection.

Heart. Diabetes can increase risk for heart disease by as much as fourfold.

Hands. Diabetes can damage nerves and blood vessels in the hands, leading to pain, tingling, numbness, and sometimes even tissue damage requiring amputation.

persuade cells to open up to glucose, which it does by creating tiny doorways on cell walls that allow glucose to enter. In people with diabetes, however, this doesn't happen. Either the pancreas fails to provide insulin in the first place, which constitutes type 1 diabetes, or the body's cells don't respond to insulin even if it is produced, which constitutes the far more common type 2 form of the disease.

Either way, the end result is pretty much the same: Glucose builds up in the blood, and cells, paradoxically, go hungry despite the excess.

Kidneys. Kidney failure is more common in people with diabetes by a margin of twentyfold.

Stomach. Nausea, vomiting, constipation, or diarrhea can result from a condition called *gastroparesis* caused when diabetes damages nerves in the stomach responsible for normal digestion.

Bladder. People with diabetes are more susceptible to bladder infections and urinary incontinence.

Sex organs. The nerve damage and blood flow restriction characteristic of diabetes can lead to sexual dysfunction in both sexes.

Legs. Muscular weakness and atrophy can result as diabetes causes a condition known as intermittent claudication that severely reduces blood flow.

Feet. Foot infections of all types are more common in people with diabetes, some of which can lead to amputation if not properly treated in time.

INSULT TO INJURY: KETOACIDOSIS

Elevated glucose can do more than make the blood "sticky." High blood sugar levels can lead to a potentially life-threatening condition known as *ketoacidosis*, which results when the body has to resort to burning fat instead of glucose as an energy source. The reason diabetes makes glucose levels rise in the blood in the first place, remember, is that glucose is not getting into the body's cells as it should. This forces

Gluttons for Glucose

Glucose, also called blood sugar, enters the blood from the small intestine after being converted by the process of digestion from the food we eat. By way of the bloodstream, glucose molecules travel throughout the entire body to every cell we have, serving as the fuel for all of our vital life processes. It's not just our taste buds that have a sweet tooth, you might say, but also our hearts, lungs, muscles, nerves, eyes, ears, and brains. Our brains are our greatest glucose gluttons of all, in fact, using, with the help of the rest of the central nervous system, a hefty 9 tablespoons of glucose every day. Even blood cells need glucose—about 3 tablespoons a day.

In addition to making glucose from the food we eat, however, we also store glucose in a form called *glycogen* in our livers and even our muscles, and we can store quite a lot. Marathon runners, as an example, can store almost enough glucose (about 300 grams, or a little more than 10 ounces) to transport them 26.2 miles to the finish line before having to switch over to burning fat. That's pretty good mileage for a fuel that doesn't even need its own tank but instead just fits in where it can.

As miraculous, vital, and readily available as glucose is, however, it suffers from just one drawback, and it's because of this drawback that diabetes can begin to take root. Glucose cannot work alone. Like a lock needs a key, glucose needs insulin, a hormone produced by the pancreas. Insulin works to unlock tiny doors on cell walls (called *insulin receptor sites*) that allow glucose to enter and work its energizing magic. But in people with diabetes, unfortunately, insulin is not always produced in sufficient amounts, or cells have lost their ability to "open up" to it as they should.

the body to resort to burning a much less desirable fuel—namely, molecules of fat in the blood—so that the body can continue to function. When fat is burned, however, it creates highly acidic by-products called *ketones*, and these can begin to have corrosive effects on blood vessel walls as well as the organs to which the ketones circulate.

The buildup of these ketones does not usually reach an acute stage in people with type 2 diabetes, because in this form of the disease there is usually at least *some* insulin available, and insulin helps prevent ketone formation by keeping fat molecules inside the body's fat cells where it can't be metabolized so easily. But in type 1 diabetes, in which little or no insulin is available, these ketones can become a problem, and a potentially very serious one. Signs that ketoacidosis is developing include:

> *H*igh blood sugar levels can lead to a potentially life-threatening condition known as ketoacidosis, *which results when the body has to resort to burning fat instead of glucose as an energy source.*

Abdominal pain	Nausea
Blurred vision	Rapid breathing
Flushed face	Sweet-smelling breath
Mental confusion	Vomiting

All are signs that medical attention should be sought immediately because coma and even death can result if the condition is allowed to persist for more than just a few hours. An estimated 75,000 people are hospitalized for ketoacidosis every year, and approximately 4,000 people die from the condition.

TYPE 1 VERSUS TYPE 2: A CLOSER LOOK

If you're still a bit confused about the differences between type 1 and type 2 diabetes, don't feel bad. Although their causes are different, their symptoms can be very similar, as we'll be seeing in a moment.

Just remember that while people with type 1 diabetes usually do not produce any insulin at all, and therefore must receive daily insulin injections, people with the far more common type 2 form of diabetes usually *do* produce insulin, but the problem is that their bodies have lost the ability to respond to it. The result is *too much* insulin in the blood as the pancreas often will begin to overproduce the hormone in its attempt to keep blood sugar under control.

This overproduction of insulin can begin to create problems in its own right, as insulin helps the body store extra calories as fat, thus setting into motion a vicious cycle by contributing to the very obesity that often is instrumental in the onset of type 2 diabetes in the first place.

Type 1

Type 1 diabetes constitutes only 5 to 10 percent of all cases, but it can be the more problematic kind because the pancreas fails to produce any usable insulin at all. More common in whites than other racial groups, type 1 diabetes usually develops suddenly—often within just a few weeks, in fact—and usually strikes during childhood. (Half of all people diagnosed with type 1 diabetes are under the age of 20 while type 2 is most common in—although certainly not restricted to—people over the age of 45.)

> *Type 1 diabetes usually develops suddenly—often within just a few weeks, in fact—and usually strikes during childhood.*

Also unusual about type 1 diabetes is that it's an *autoimmune disease*—a disorder caused by the body itself. It develops when the body's normally functioning immune system mistakenly interprets insulin-producing beta cells in the pancreas as harmful and destroys them as it would a legitimate threat. Exactly why this happens is still under investigation, but prime suspects—as we'll be looking at more closely shortly—include genetic influences, viruses, and molecular misfits known as *free radicals*.

People first developing type 1 diabetes may experience abdominal pain and vomiting, and sometimes they are thought to be suffering from appendicitis or the flu as a result. At the greatest risk for developing type 1 diabetes are people with a history of the disease in their families.

Type 2

Type 2 diabetes is responsible for an estimated 90 to 95 percent of all cases, and although it shares many of the same symptoms as type 1 diabetes, it differs in that it tends to be slow in making itself known. While type 1 can develop as quickly as within just a few weeks, for example, type 2 can take years and even decades, producing symptoms at rates that can differ according to the reasons for its onset. In some cases, as mentioned earlier, the pancreas produces insulin but not enough. In other cases, the pancreas produces enough insulin, but the insulin is not of sufficient quality. In still other cases, the pancreas does its job of producing insulin of adequate quantity as well quality, but the problem lies with the body's cells, which have lost their ability

---

Type 1 Diabetes

Most common symptoms:
- Abdominal pain, nausea, or vomiting
- Excessive hunger
- Excessive thirst
- Fatigue
- Frequent urination
- Irritability
- Weakness
- Weight loss

Greatest risk factor:
- Having a history of the disease in the family

to "open up" to the insulin as they should. This leaves excess glucose to wander through the bloodstream as if the pancreas had produced no insulin at all.

Then, too, there can be combinations of all of these factors, making type 2 diabetes a very complex problem indeed. And a very prevalent one. While type 1 diabetes has been increasing moderately in recent years, type 2 diabetes has been skyrocketing, possibly because its two greatest risk factors—obesity and lack of exercise—also have been increasing at an alarming rate. Other risk factors for type 2 diabetes include age (it's most common in people 45 and older), a family history of the disease, and low levels of HDL cholesterol or high levels of triglycerides (fats) in the blood. Certain ethnic or racial groups also show higher incidence of type 2 diabetes (including African Americans, Latinos, Asians, Pacific Islanders, and Native Americans) and women who have had gestational diabetes or have given birth to a baby weighing 9 pounds or more are also at an increased risk for developing the disease.

> *Although type 2 diabetes shares many of the same symptoms of type 1 diabetes, it differs in that it tends to be slow in making itself known.*

OTHER TYPES, SIMILAR GRIPES

Although an estimated 95 percent of all cases of diabetes are either type 1 or 2, other types exist as well. All have the same basic problem in common, however, which is a failure of glucose to be adequately absorbed by the body's cells, leading to potentially harmful accumulations in the blood.

Gestational Diabetes

This type of diabetes is brought on by pregnancy, and while only 2 to 5 percent of pregnant women ever develop it, and it usually ends following birth, women who do contract gestational diabetes are at increased risk for developing type 2 diabetes later in life. The symptoms

Type 2 Diabetes

As mentioned, symptoms of type 2 diabetes tend to be the same as those of type 1 (see page 13), but may include the following as well.

Most common symptoms
(in addition to those listed for type 1):
- Blurred vision
- Cuts and bruises that are slow to heal
- Frequent infections, especially of the skin, gums, or bladder
- Tingling or numbness in the hands or feet

Greatest risk factors:
- Being more than 20 percent overweight
- Being 45 years of age or older
- Having high blood pressure
- Having high blood fats (triglycerides and LDL cholesterol)
- Being of African American, Native American, Asian, Hispanic, or Pacific Island descent
- Being a woman who has had gestational diabetes
- Being a woman who has had a baby weighing more than 9 pounds at birth
- Having a parent or sibling with the disease

of gestational diabetes generally are similar to those of type 2 diabetes, and they are thought to be due to chemical imbalances caused by hormones produced by the placenta, the protective membrane in which the baby develops. These hormones can block the normal action of insulin in the mother's body, resulting in high glucose levels just as with types 1 and 2. The weight gain associated with pregnancy also can lead to insulin resistance, thus compounding whatever insulin resistance may be hormonal. (Pregnancy, even in women without gestational diabetes, can increase insulin needs by as much as threefold.)

Although gestational diabetes does not pose the same risks for birth defects as when a pregnant women has either type 1 or 2, it can pose dangers to the fetus if not controlled. This is because high blood sugar levels in the mom cross the placenta and cause high blood sugar levels in the baby. This in turn causes the baby to produce more insulin, which can convert the baby's extra blood sugar into fat, increasing risks of obesity both at birth and later in life. Because a baby's obesity also can make the birthing process itself difficult, damage to the baby's shoulders can occur if birth is natural, often making cesarean section the preferred method of delivery when fetal obesity has developed. Other problems that can occur in the baby after birth when the mother has gestational diabetes include breathing difficulties, low calcium and magnesium levels, and low blood sugar, as the baby usually will continue to produce large amounts of insulin for several hours even after the maternal supply of glucose has ceased.

While only 2 to 5 percent of pregnant women ever develop gestational diabetes and it usually ends following birth, women who do contract it are at increased risk for developing type 2 diabetes later in life.

All of these potential complications point to the importance of catching gestational diabetes early, before it can set such events into motion, which is why screening for the disorder is recommended between weeks 24 and 28 during pregnancy. The risk for gestational diabetes is greatest if the mother is:

- Age 25 or older
- Overweight before becoming pregnant
- From a family with a history of diabetes
- Hispanic, African American, Native American, or of Asian or Pacific Island descent

If discovered, gestational diabetes should be treated immediately with a combination of dietary changes, physical activity, and sometimes insulin (and all under the supervision of the appropriate health care team, of course.) To prevent future blood sugar problems, moreover, women who develop gestational diabetes should have their blood sugar levels checked 6 weeks after delivery and, even if blood sugar levels are normal, at least once every 3 years after that.

Other Forms of Diabetes

In rare circumstances, other forms of diabetes can develop in response to specific problems such as genetic abnormalities, surgeries, drug side effects, malnutrition, infections, and illnesses. The basic problem with these other types is always the same as with types 1 and 2 and gestational diabetes: a failure of the body to metabolize glucose adequately.

NO EFFORT TOO SMALL

The recent escalation of type 2 diabetes—and among younger age groups, especially—is certainly alarming. But in the darkness of the cloud should be seen the glimmer of a brighter lining: Diabetes can do its greatest harm *only when it's allowed to*, and this goes for its short-term and long-term complications alike.

Currently as many as 50 percent of all people with diabetes may not even know they have it. This is dangerous as well as unfortunate because it allows complications to develop that otherwise might not. And much like cancer, diabetes is a disease best caught as early as possible to minimize its long-term risks. We'll be looking more closely at the importance of early diagnosis in chapter 2, but it certainly can't hurt to make the point here as well: With diabetes, it's the "early bird" who gets the health.

The following list of potential complications associated with diabetes should be viewed with that point in mind. The sooner diabetes

Type 1 or Type 2?

While type 1 and type 2 diabetes result from the same basic problem—namely, the buildup of harmful levels of blood sugar (glucose)
in the bloodstream due to an inability of the body's cells to use
and/or produce insulin—how that glucose gets there, and why, can
be very different. Here are the primary distinctions between the two
major types of this disease:

- The onset of type 1 diabetes usually occurs suddenly and is
  marked by extreme thirst, excessive appetite, frequent urination, and debilitating fatigue. Type 2, on the other hand, may
  involve similar symptoms, but the symptoms usually develop
  slowly and may be difficult to notice at all in milder cases.

- While type 1 diabetes usually strikes before the age of 20,
  type 2 usually does not develop until after the age of 40.

- While people with type 1 diabetes tend to be lean when diagnosed, people with type 2 usually are overweight, especially
  in the area of the abdomen.

- Type 1 diabetes is an autoimmune disease caused by destruction of insulin-producing cells within the pancreas by the
  body's immune system, but type 2 is thought to be a disease
  brought on more by lifestyle conditions such as obesity and

is diagnosed and the better it's managed, the less likely any of these
problems will occur. And even if problems do occur, effort is still the
key. Keeping blood sugar levels as normal as possible—whether
through diet, exercise, medication, or all three—can make the difference between good health and ill health regardless of how far the disease has progressed.

lack of exercise. With both types, however, a predisposition to developing the disease may be inherited.

- While people with type 1 diabetes require daily insulin injections, people with type 2 frequently do not. Often they can keep their glucose levels under control by making lifestyle changes such as modifying their diets, losing weight, and being more physically active.

- Long-term complications of type 1 diabetes most often involve the small blood vessels of the eyes, kidneys, and nerves, while the most common long-term problems associated with type 2 tend to involve the larger blood vessels of the arms, legs, hands, feet, and heart. (Type 1 can also do large blood vessel damage, however, just as type 2 can also do small blood vessel harm.)

- While type 1 diabetes is most common among whites, type 2 is most prevalent among African Americans, Native Americans, Hispanics, and people of Pacific Island and Asian descent. Type 2 also appears to be the more "inheritable" of the two diseases, as evidenced by studies with identical twins: While the chance that an identical twin of someone with type 1 diabetes will have the disease is 25 to 50 percent, for example, the odds increase to 60 to 75 percent with type 2.

Support for that advice lies in a 10-year study of more than 1,400 people with diabetes, as reported in *The American Diabetes Association Complete Guide To Diabetes*. The Diabetes Control and Complications Trial, published in 1993, found that patients who did the most to control their diabetes without question got the most benefit back. Compared to a group of patients that was more lax about controlling blood sugar levels, the diligent group suffered 76 percent less eye disease, 60 percent less nerve damage, and between 35 and 56 percent less kidney damage in return for their efforts. The people in the study had type 1 diabetes, but the researchers expressed confidence that similar results could have been achieved with type 2 patients as well.

> *Keeping blood sugar levels as normal as possible can make the difference between good health and ill health regardless of how far diabetes has progressed.*

Better yet, the battle against the ill effects of diabetes doesn't have to be an all-or-nothing affair. Yes, greater effort grants greater rewards, but it's comforting to know, too, that any effort that's put toward controlling blood sugar levels is vastly better than none at all. When it comes to minimizing symptoms of both types of the disease, the bottom line is very clear: The less time the body has to contend with too much glucose in the blood, the better. Nor is it ever "too late" to get efforts to control the disease started. "Most conditions can be helped by improving blood glucose control even if they have already developed," the American Diabetes Association says.

WHAT CAN GO WRONG

As discouraging as some of these potential complications might seem, keep in mind that perhaps more than any other disease, diabetes is an illness that *we* have the power to control. Eating better, exercising regularly, and taking the appropriate medications can reduce the disease from a roar to little more than a whimper.

Short-Term Complications: Warnings of Worse to Come

The most common short-term complications of diabetes should be seen as warning signs that longer-term and more serious consequences may be around the bend if appropriate treatment and methods of control are not pursued. These warning signs may include the following:

- **Fatigue, muscular weakness, and mental confusion** as the buildup of glucose in the blood means that the glucose is not getting to the body's muscle, nerve, and brain cells as it should

- **Excessive urination followed by excessive thirst** and possibly dehydration as the body must draw fluid from wherever it can to help minimize glucose accumulation as best it can

- **Weight loss** despite seemingly constant hunger as glucose lost in the urine means glucose—and hence calories—are not being absorbed by the body

> *Eating better, exercising regularly, and taking the appropriate medications can reduce the disease from a roar to little more than a whimper.*

LONG-TERM RISKS: THE DANGERS THAT DON'T HAVE TO BE

What other, longer-term complications can develop as a consequence of diabetes? Because high levels of glucose in the blood are circulated throughout the body, the long-term risks posed by diabetes can be extensive, as the following sections show. Earlier detection and better management of diabetes could lessen its impact dramatically, however, so please view these potential complications with that point well in mind. The results of several newly completed studies make it clear that diabetes is not a disease of destiny, after all, and that its effects usually can be minimized according to the amount of effort a patient is willing to invest in keeping the condition under control.

Cardiovascular Disease

People with diabetes have two to four times the risk of suffering from a heart attack and five times the risk of having a stroke as people without the disease, and a quick look inside the body's arteries should show why: The high glucose levels associated with diabetes can make whatever cholesterol or triglycerides that may be in the blood more likely to stick to artery walls, clogging them and restricting blood flow. This is why it's especially important for people with diabetes to control their fat intake as they keep their glucose levels in check, because the two can be a deadly duo indeed. If an artery to the heart becomes seriously obstructed, a heart attack can result; if an artery to the brain becomes clogged, a stroke can occur. Blockages in arteries to the legs can cause pain and weakness known as *intermittent claudication*. To reduce risks of cardiovascular complications, people with diabetes, in addition to controlling their blood sugar and avoiding a high-fat diet, should keep their blood pressure under control, be physically active, avoid smoking, and maintain a healthy weight.

> *The high glucose levels associated with diabetes can make whatever cholesterol or triglycerides that may be in the blood more likely to stick to artery walls, clogging them and restricting blood flow.*

High Blood Pressure

Anyone can have high blood pressure (hypertension), but the condition is more common in people with diabetes, and type 2 diabetes, especially. An estimated 60 percent of the latter group have hypertension, a condition marked by the buildup of undue pressure as blood cannot move as freely as it should through the body's vascular network. It's especially important for diabetics to control their blood pressure (levels of 135/85 or below are recommended) because high levels can further increase already-elevated risks for heart disease, strokes, eye problems, and kidney disease.

Many medications are available for controlling hypertension, but people with diabetes need to be careful to avoid those that may interfere with the glucose-lowering action of insulin. Losing weight, exercising regularly, and—in people who are sodium-sensitive—restricting sodium intake can help many of these individuals keep their blood pressure within normal limits.

Eye Problems

The delicacy of the membranes of the eyes makes them a prime target for the tissue-damaging effects of diabetes, and the statistics show it: Diabetes currently is the leading cause of blindness in people ages 20 to 74, with between 12,000 and 24,000 people losing their sight to the disease annually. The most common problem is known as *retinopathy*, which causes vision to be blurred as blood vessels to the retina (the light-sensing portion of the eye) either rupture or become blocked. If left untreated, the condition can progress to a more serious problem known as *proliferative retinopathy* in which new blood vessels sprout within the eye, only to rupture easily, causing fluid to leak into the portion of the eye in front of the retina. This condition can impair vision further as scar tissue develops, and if the scar tissue begins to shrink, it can cause blindness by tearing the layers of the retina apart. Retinopathy also can lead to a condition called *macular edema*, a swelling of the central portion of the retina responsible for seeing in fine detail.

The delicacy of the membranes of the eyes makes them a target for tissue-damaging effects of diabetes.

Because such problems frequently can be successfully treated if detected early, it's important for people with diabetes to have their eyes checked often. All people with diabetes ages 30 or older should have an eye exam every year, as should patients regardless of age if they've had their disease for 5 years or longer. In the Diabetes Control and Complications Trial, retinopathy and other eye conditions were found to be the most preventable of all diabetic problems—down by 76 percent in the group most diligent about their glucose control.

Kidney Disease

Called *nephropathy*, kidney disease affects one-third of people with type 1 diabetes and 10 to 20 percent of people with type 2 after 15 years.

But again, tighter glucose control could no doubt bring these numbers down. Diabetes damages the kidneys by causing the small blood vessels within the organ not just to become blocked, but to leak, thus compromising the organ's ability to do its highly important job of clearing the blood of potentially harmful toxins. The damage also causes the body to lose protein and other valuable nutrients in the urine.

As with eye problems, the good news is that diligent glucose control can lessen the risks of kidney disease substantially.

Symptoms of kidney damage (weakness, fatigue, and sometimes vomiting) usually don't appear until as much as 80 percent of the organ has been destroyed, unfortunately, but as with eye problems, the good news is that diligent glucose control can lessen the risks of kidney disease substantially. Coupled with efforts to control high blood pressure (also very damaging to the delicate blood vessels within the kidneys), keeping blood sugar levels in check can reduce the risks of kidney damage by over 50 percent.

Nerve Damage

Roughly half of all people with diabetes will have some type of nerve damage (called *neuropathy*) after 25 years. Prolonged periods of high glucose levels in the blood can begin to damage the tiny blood vessels that nerves rely on for oxygen and other nutrients. Making matters worse, high glucose levels also can begin to erode the layer of fat that protects nerves like the rubber coating around an electrical wire. Without this protective coating, or enough oxygen and nutrients, nerves affected by diabetes can lose their ability to function, often causing pain as they do. The result is a "double whammy" that can lead to a wide variety of problems depending on where the nerve damage has occurred.

Again, however, the good news is that people with diabetes who closely monitor their glucose levels, compared to those who do not, should be able to reduce their nerve damage by as much as 60 percent. (See the sidebar, "Nerves Unnerved," for a more detailed look at the specific conditions such monitoring is likely to deter.)

Infections

Chronically high glucose levels, as we've seen, can interfere with many of the body's most important functions—and resistance to infection, unfortunately, is one of them. The excess blood sugar characteristic of diabetes not only renders white blood cells less effective at killing bacteria and viruses, but also can give certain germs added vigor as they feed on the glucose for fuel. As a result, people with diabetes tend to have more infections virtually everywhere in their bodies—from the mouth and gums clear down to the feet. Not even the genital area or bladder is exempt, and even minor surgeries can become major infection risks.

> *The excess blood sugar characteristic of diabetes not only renders white blood cells less effective at killing bacteria and viruses, but also can give certain germs added vigor.*

Worse yet, numbness in certain areas of the body caused by diabetic nerve damage can lessen sensitivity to injuries such as minor cuts or burns, thus increasing the chances of their going unnoticed and breeding infections the diabetic body has decreased powers to fight. The healing of wounds can be hampered, too, since diabetes frequently leads to partial blockage of blood vessels and a slowing of blood needed to bring healing nutrients to the injured areas. We take a closer look shortly at one of the areas of the body most vulnerable to infection in people with diabetes—the feet.

CURABLE, NO; MANAGEABLE, ABSOLUTELY

As with all serious diseases, the hope for a cure for diabetes springs eternal, and while scientists remain encouraged with their research into new medications and surgical techniques such as pancreas-cell transplants, the bulk of the responsibility for controlling diabetes still

Nerves Unnerved

Perhaps no other problems caused by diabetes are as exasperating as those involving the nervous system, and for a very simple reason: The nervous system does so much. Its incredibly intricate network of intercommunicating chemicals and cells is responsible for everything we see, taste, hear, touch, and even think, so it's no wonder we can feel out of sorts if a glitch occurs. And diabetes, unfortunately, can cause such glitches in many different ways. We'll be looking at these in more detail but here's a quick look at the three basic parts of the nervous system most likely to be affected and a sneak preview of some of things that most commonly go wrong.

Peripheral Nervous System Problems

Most diabetic nerve problems involve the peripheral nervous system, which includes the nerves of the arms, legs, hands, feet, abdomen, and back. Symptoms usually are most pronounced at night and can range from mild tingling and numbness to sharp stabs of needlelike pain or even sensations that some sufferers describe as feeling like electrical shocks. Sometimes accompanied by muscular weakness, pain may be symmetrical, affecting both sides of the body equally, or asymmetrical, affecting one side only. Pain involving the peripheral nerves of the abdomen or chest may mimic other medical conditions such as heart attack, kidney stones, or appendicitis and hence may require a test known as an *electromylogram* (EMG) to be correctly diagnosed. Fortunately, the worst pains involving the peripheral nervous system rarely last longer than a few months.

rests with the people who have it—and with the people they rely on for support. This means not just loved ones and family members, but also the health care providers responsible for assisting diabetic patients in their management efforts. It truly is a team effort that's needed to tame this disease.

Cranial Nervous System Problems

The cranial nerves include those that go to the face, eyes, ears, and jaw, and these, too, can be adversely affected by high glucose levels. When the nerves to the muscles of the eyes are damaged, the eyes may fail to move in unison, causing double vision. The problem usually is only temporary, however, and usually corrects itself in a matter of several months, leaving no permanent damage.

Also usually temporary is another problem called Bell's palsy, which can develop when diabetes damages one of the nerves that controls the muscles of the face. Typically one of the eyelids will droop as will the corner of the mouth on the same side, but it's rare for the condition to cause any permanent problems.

Autonomic Nervous System Problems

The autonomic nervous system controls the workings of the internal organs, including the heart, stomach, intestines, and even blood vessels. The effects of damage to this system depend on which organ has been harmed and to what degree. Damage to the nerves controlling the stomach, for example, can lead to a condition known as *gastroparesis,* which can cause the stomach to empty very slowly, sometimes causing nausea or vomiting. If diabetes affects the nerves of the intestines, constipation or diarrhea may result. Damage to the nerves of the bladder can interfere with the ability to know it's "time to go," thus increasing risks of urinary tract infections, and damage to the nerves of the sex organs can lead to loss of feeling and function in men and women alike.

As experts in the field are eager to point out, however, the measures needed to control diabetes are no different from the measures all of us should be pursuing for good health—eating a nutritious, low-fat, high-fiber diet; being physically active; and controlling our weight. Anyone with diabetes might view their disease as an advantage, in fact, in that it adds incentive for them to adhere to the same health strategies we all should adopt. The latest research (including the previously mentioned Diabetes Control and Complications Trial and the more recent Finnish Diabetes Prevention Study) makes it comfortingly clear that if the effort is there, the results can be, too.

> *The measures needed to control diabetes are no different from the measures all of us should be pursuing for good health—eating a nutritious, low-fat, high-fiber diet; being physically active; and controlling our weight.*

CAUSES

Although diabetes has been under medical investigation since the time of the ancient Egyptians, its causes still remain largely unknown. Yes, we know that excess glucose builds up in the blood due either to a lack of insulin (as in type 1) or a failure of insulin to get glucose into the body's cells (as in type 2), but the reasons these problems occur in the first place are still being sought. Researchers continue to work diligently to better understand the disease, however, and more pieces to the puzzle are being discovered all the time. Here's a quick rundown of what's been found so far and also what's being theorized about the causes of this so common yet confounding disease.

Type 1 Diabetes

Here are the theories currently at the top of the leaderboard concerning the mechanisms that may give type 1 diabetes its start:

- **Autoimmunity: When the Body "Bites" Itself.** While much of what causes type 1 diabetes remains uncertain, scientists do know that the illness qualifies as an autoimmune disease, which means it's caused by a mistake in the functioning of the body's immune system. Other conditions are known to be autoimmune diseases—multiple sclerosis, lupus, and certain thyroid illnesses such as Grave's disease, for example—and what they have in common is that innocent cells get destroyed by an all-too-vigilant immune system that erroneously interprets them as potentially harmful invaders. The cells that are destroyed in type 1 diabetes are the all-important insulin-producing beta cells located in the pancreas, a destruction that usually takes place during childhood, leaving the body with no way to get glucose properly metabolized for energy and other vital processes. The big question—as with all autoimmune diseases, of course—is "Why?" And while scientists don't yet have a definite answer, they do have some suspicions.

- **Genetics.** One needs a diagnostic tool no more sophisticated than the family tree to show there's a genetic component to type 1 diabetes. The disease is definitely more common in children of parents afflicted with the disorder, as well as in certain racial groups. Whites, for example, are more likely to get the disease than African Americans, Native Americans, or Hispanics, and while researchers have not yet identified any one gene responsible, they have narrowed their search down to several. This gives scientists hope that in the future it may be possible to identify people carrying any of these "susceptibility genes" before the disease strikes, thus allowing preventive treatments to be started before any irreparable damage to the body's insulin-producing cells has been done.

> *Diabetes qualifies as an autoimmune disease, which means it's caused by a mistake in the functioning of the body's immune system.*

- **Viruses.** The theory that viruses may cause type 1 diabetes has arisen from the observation that huge increases in the disease frequently have occurred following outbreaks of viral diseases such as mumps and German measles. This observation has led

to research suggesting that certain viruses—particularly those
of one family known as the Coxsackie family—may cause the
disease not directly but rather indirectly by posing as "look-
alikes" to insulin-producing beta cells. After the body's immune
system has taught its virus-killing T cells to destroy the
Coxsackie viruses, therefore, these cells may go on to kill the
beta cells as well. Another theory holds that invading viruses
might simply alter beta cells directly in ways that make them
appear to be foreign to the body, thus making them subject to
immune system attack. And lastly, the Italian researcher Gian
Franco Botazzo, based on sudden outbreaks of type 1 diabetes
in Italy in the 1960s and Finland in the 1970s, has proposed
that the disorder is a relatively recent condition caused by a
slow-acting virus that causes the immune system gradually to
destroy proteins in the pancreas responsible for adequate insulin output.

- **Free Radicals.** They sound nasty, and they are. *Free radicals*
  are molecules in the body formed as by-products of normal
  metabolic processes, but they can do harm if allowed to reach
  abnormally high levels due to such unhealthful influences as
  smoking, air pollution, or even just a shoddy diet. Normally
  the body has enzymes to neutralize these troublemakers, but
  research shows that the cells within the pancreas responsible
  for producing insulin have relatively low levels of these protective enzymes and hence may be especially vulnerable to free
  radical attack.

- **Chemicals and Drugs.** A chemical compound used in rat poison,
  pyriminil (Vacor), has been found to trigger type 1 diabetes, as
  have two prescription drugs: pentamidine, used to treat pneumonia, and L-asparaginase, an enzyme used to treat cancer. Other
  chemicals have been shown to make laboratory animals diabetic,
  but uncertainty remains regarding their effects on humans.

- **Cow's Milk for Infants.** The link by no means has been confirmed but should be mentioned, nonetheless. Some research has suggested that feeding cow's milk to infants prior to the age of 3 or 4 months may increase the risk of type 1 diabetes, but other research has failed to duplicate the findings. Further study will be needed before any connection between cow's milk and the development of type 1 diabetes can be established.

> *Cells within the pancreas responsible for producing insulin have relatively low levels of the protective enzymes to neutralize free radicals and hence may be especially vulnerable to free radical attack.*

Type 2 Diabetes

While the causes of faulty insulin production and insulin resistance in type 2 diabetes is still not entirely understood, scientists do know what factors can increase type 2 risks:

- **Genetics.** As with type 1 diabetes, one's parents may have as much to do with the onset of type 2 diabetes as anything else. If one parent has type 2 diabetes, for example, the odds of the disease being passed to an offspring are one in seven. If both parents have the disease, the chances increase to one in two. Yet this does not mean that one's diabetic destiny is clinched at the time of birth. In both type 1 and type 2 diabetes, "two factors are important," says the ADA. "First, you must inherit a predisposition to diabetes. Second, something in the environment must trigger the disease."

- **Obesity.** So closely linked are body weight and type 2 diabetes that some clever clinician has coined the term "diabesity." Being obese (defined as being more than 20 percent above ideal weight; see the "At-Risk Weight Chart" on page 40) seems not only to reduce the number of insulin receptor cites on cells but to cause changes inside cells that make them more resistant to insulin as well.

But perhaps even more important than the number of extra pounds we carry is *where* we carry them. Fat in the region of the abdomen appears to pose a far greater risk for type 2 diabetes than extra weight carried in the area of the hips or thighs. It's more dangerous to be shaped like an apple, in other words, than a pear. Why this is true, however, still remains unclear. But what is known is the magnitude of the risk that obesity entails:

> *It's more dangerous to be shaped like an apple than a pear.*

In a study of more than 8,000 people conducted by David Williamson, Ph.D., of the Centers for Disease Control and Prevention in Atlanta, it was found that the risk for developing type 2 diabetes increased by 9 percent for every extra pound carried. A little grade-school math will show you that a mere 10 pounds over one's ideal weight means that the risk for type 2 diabetes goes up by nearly 100 percent.

- **Lack of Exercise.** Lack of exercise may not increase the risk of type 2 diabetes directly, but it can certainly do so indirectly by encouraging weight gain. Once type 2 diabetes has developed, however, there's no question that regular exercise can lessen both the severity of the disease as well as any insulin that may be required. This is because exercise increases the body's sensitivity to whatever insulin is available in addition to using up glucose in its own right, as glucose is needed to fuel the exercising muscles. Depending on intensity, glucose uptake can increase by as much as seven- to twentyfold during a 30 to 40 minute exercise session, reports David C. Nieman, Dr.PH., in his book *The Exercise Health Connection*. Dr. Nieman reports that some people with type 2 diabetes taking insulin who lose weight and exercise regularly are able to eliminate their needs for the medication entirely. And while there has been some concern that exercise may increase the risk of heart attack in people with type 2 diabetes because they usually have other risk factors for infarction, one study of more than 500 patients done at the University of Pittsburgh showed that regular physical activity had just the opposite effect by extending their life spans.

- **Diet.** Is it possible to cause diabetes by eating a diet too high in sugar? As with lack of exercise, the link is indirect rather than direct, says the American Diabetes Association. A diet high in sugar is also apt to be high in calories and hence apt to cause weight gain, and being overweight definitely can contribute to the development of type 2 diabetes. "Whether the excess pounds are from eating candy or bagels or meat loaf," however, "makes little difference," the ADA reports.

- **Age.** While type 1 diabetes is definitely a disease of youth, striking most sufferers during their childhood or as young adults, type 2 diabetes has a target audience of people 45 or older. But as with activity levels and diet, the real reason type 2 diabetes becomes more common as we age may

> *Dr. Nieman reports that some people with type 2 diabetes taking insulin who lose weight and exercise regularly are able to eliminate their needs for the medication entirely.*

simply be that we tend also to become more plump. Fully 50 percent of all new cases of type 2 diabetes are diagnosed in people over 55, the ADA reports, yet many researchers think the reason is not so much our advancing years as our advancing waistlines, the group hastens to add. Our tendency to reduce our activity levels as we mature no doubt contributes to our burgeoning bellies and hence diabetes risks as well.

DIABETIC FOR A DAY

So what's it actually like to have diabetes? That depends not just on the type and severity of the disease, but also on the degree to which the illness is being controlled, and not just day to day, but hour to hour. Some people with very serious cases of diabetes who are diligent about monitoring their blood sugar levels may suffer fewer consequences than patients with less severe conditions who are lax in their blood sugar control. The disease might be considered "fair," in other words, in that it rewards hard work.

Carol, for example, a 53-year-old supermarket checkout clerk who was diagnosed with type 2 diabetes 10 years ago, admits that how she feels is pretty much her choice to make. "If I follow my meal plan and take my pills when I should, I feel fine. But if I don't, I pay for it. When my sugar gets too high, I begin to feel tired and get thirsty and feel weak. And it doesn't take long. If I miss taking my pills by just a few hours, I can feel the effects."

Our tendency to reduce our activity levels as we mature no doubt contributes to our burgeoning bellies and hence diabetes risks as well.

The condition Carol is describing is called *hyperglycemia*—the prefix *hyper* meaning "high" and *glycemia* meaning "sugar in the blood." Besides fatigue and thirst, symptoms of hyperglycemia also can include nausea, diarrhea, facial flushing, and rapid breathing. People with diabetes, especially those with type 1, need to be particularly careful to avoid hyperglycemia during times of emotional distress or physical illness, both of which can increase the body's needs for insulin. Insulin needs can increase so much during times of emotional duress or physical illness, in fact, that even people with type 2 diabetes who do not normally require insulin sometimes need the hormone to get glucose levels back to where they should be.

But Carol also can have a bad day if she skips a meal or is especially active, thus causing a condition known as *hypoglycemia*, *hypo* meaning "low." Also known as "insulin shock," the problem is far more common with type 1 diabetes, but it can occur with type 2 patients if they go too long without eating or have been especially active. The symptoms of hypoglycemia can include feeling dizzy, light-headed, shaky, sweaty, or suddenly very hungry. If food is not eaten and glucose levels

The Ethnicity Factor

For reasons not fully understood, certain ethnic groups are more prone to develop type 2 diabetes than others. Here, according to the American Diabetes Association, is how the disease breaks down according to ethnic categories. Percentages, in most cases, represent prevalence of the disease in people ages 45 to 74.

White Americans: 6 percent

African Americans: 10 percent

Asian Americans and Pacific Islanders: 12 percent

Native Americans: 12 percent (some tribes, 50 percent)

Cuban Americans: 16 percent

Mexican Americans: 24 percent

Puerto Rican Americans: 26 percent

continue to drop, these initial symptoms can progress to headache, blurred vision, numbness or tingling of the lips, a pale complexion, or mental confusion. In severe cases, loss of consciousness, brain damage, and even death can occur, so it's not a condition to be taken lightly. Usually eating a snack high in carbohydrates can correct hypoglycemia within 15 to 20 minutes, but in emergency situations, a prescription medication called *glucagon* may be required. Needless to say, it's best not to let hypoglycemia develop in the first place.

"But my biggest concern right now," Carol says, "is getting disability insurance in case my condition gets so bad I can't work. Mainly it's the numbness in my hands I'm worried about, because when it gets bad I can have trouble operating the register."

Physical hardships aside, diabetes can produce emotional strains ranging from anger and denial to depression and even guilt. In Carol's case, for example, she knows her condition would improve if she lost weight, but "food is one of my greatest pleasures," she says. "I'm afraid if I went on a strict diet I'd get really depressed, so I'm trying to cut back on my eating gradually, and I'm trying to be more active, to see if I can lose some weight that way, too. My doctor keeps telling me any progress I make is a lot better than nothing, so that's been a help. Basically I just try to take things one day at a time."

A SHORT HISTORY OF DIABETES: FROM ANTHILLS TO INSULIN

We tend to think of diabetes as a disease as modern as the junk foods and TV clickers that can encourage its onset, yet an ancient Egyptian manuscript known as the Ebers Papyrus describes people suffering from excessive urination and extreme thirst—two of the most common symptoms of diabetes—as long ago as 1500 B.C. These early writings even describe a diagnostic test for the disease: The urine of a suspected sufferer was poured near an anthill, and if its sugar content was sufficient to attract the hill's inhabitants, diabetes was confirmed.

The condition would not be called *diabetes*, however, until a Greek physician named Aretaeus in the second century A.D. assigned it a word that meant "to flow"—an apparent reference to his observation that sufferers of the disease seemed constantly to be doing just that in their frequent need to urinate. The sweet aroma of the urine of people with diabetes, led to the addition of the Latin word *mellitus* in the 18th century, which means "honeyed" or "sweet."

In ancient Egypt, the urine of a suspected sufferer was poured near an anthill, and if its sugar content was sufficient to attract the hill's inhabitants, diabetes was confirmed.

A cause for diabetes, however, wouldn't be suggested until 1889 when two German physiologists inadvertently induced the disease in a dog by removing the animal's pancreas as part of their work aimed at better understanding the process of human digestion. With the pancreas now targeted as a logical suspect in the etiol-

Diabetes: Some Vital Stats

What constitutes diabetes: glucose (blood sugar) levels in excess of 126 milligrams/deciliter in a fasting state or 200 milligrams/deciliter following meals

Estimated number of people in the United States who have diabetes: 16 million

Estimated number of people who have diabetes but don't know it: 5 million

Number of people who die every year from complications caused by diabetes: 200,000

Amount diabetes has increased in the general population between 1990 and 1998: 33 percent

Amount diabetes has increased in people ages 30 to 39 between 1990 and 1998: 70 percent

Average yearly medical care costs for someone with diabetes: $10,000 to $12,000

Amount diabetes costs the U.S. economy in health care costs and lost productivity every year: $98 billion

People with type 2 diabetes who are obese (20 percent or more overweight): 90 percent

People in the general population who are obese: 18 percent

Degree to which the medical complications of diabetes could be reduced if glucose levels were closely controlled: 50 percent

ogy of the disease, two Canadian researchers, Dr. Frederick Banting and Charles Best, picked up the ball in 1921 and looked further into the role played by this organ. Also working with canine rather than human subjects, Banting and Best soon discovered that a substance extracted from the pancreas, later to be called insulin, could reverse diabetic symptoms in experimental animals when injected back into their bloodstreams.

But would their extract work in a human? A 14-year-old boy who was dying from diabetes, Leonard Thompson, was elected to help the world find out. He was injected with the extract, but without results. Twelve days later, however, after the extract had been further purified, an injection was tried again and this time with great success. The emaciated boy began to gain weight immediately, and with regular injections he went on to live for another 15 years, dying not of diabetes but complications of pneumonia.

The experiment had been such a success that it earned Banting and Best the Nobel Prize for Medicine. Before long, however, it became apparent that the success had been incomplete because some patients on insulin began to reexperience their symptoms. This led to decades of more confusion over the disease, and not until 1977 would scientists finally arrive at their current understanding that there are essentially two forms of diabetes—type 1, caused by a pancreas that can't produce adequate insulin, and type 2, caused by a body that can't adequately use it.

Presently the disease is being fought successfully on both fronts as new medications continually are being developed to help the body regulate its glucose levels. Some help the pancreas increase its insulin output, while others limit the amount of glucose released into the bloodstream by the liver while also making the body's cells more insulin sensitive. Then, too, scientists have made great strides in understanding the importance of such lifestyle factors as diet, exercise, and weight loss in controlling diabetes. It all adds up to a bright future indeed.

CHAPTER 2

The Importance of Being Diagnosed

ℭℴ

Blood so thick with sugar it logjams in the body's tiniest blood vessels, depriving tissue of vital nutrients and oxygen. Nerves in the feet so squeezed by their own sugar-swollen coatings they cause pain that feels like walking on glass. And all the while, cells throughout the entire body giving up vital fluids in efforts to flush all this noxious sugar away. As we saw in chapter 1, this describes just some of the damage diabetes can do if allowed to run its ruinous course. Yet such devastation is exactly what as many as five million Americans may be risking at this very moment by having diabetes but not taking the few minutes required to get diagnosed. They're the walking wounded, the medical crises waiting to happen, and one of them could be a family member, a loved one—or even you.

In this chapter you'll learn about the simple blood tests doctors now use to test for diabetes, and you'll learn, too, about how to assemble a "dream team" of diabetes experts capable of overseeing the very best treatment possible if the disease is diagnosed. As you'll see, the best game plan for defeating diabetes includes catching it before it can get too much of a head start.

What's Your Risk? Take a Minute to Find Out

There's no question that the disability and hardship caused by diabetes could be reduced dramatically if more people would be diagnosed earlier and begin treatment in time, the experts agree. So why not try your hand at the following questions offered by the American Diabetes Association (ADA) with that in mind? The test is by no means definitive, but it can give a rough idea of the degree to which diabetes is a risk. It's especially important for African Americans, Native Americans, Asians, Hispanics, and people of Pacific Island decent to take this test, the ADA says, because diabetes is so common in these groups.

Write in the points next to each statement that is true for you. If a statement is not true, put a zero. Then add your total score.

1. I am a woman who has had a baby weighing more than nine pounds at birth.   **YES**   1   _____

2. I have a sister or brother with diabetes.   **YES**   1   _____

3. I have a parent with diabetes.   **YES**   1   _____

4. My weight is equal to or above that listed in the chart.   **YES**   5   _____

5. I am under 65 years of age **and** I get little or no exercise.   **YES**   5   _____

6. I am between 45 and 64 years of age.   **YES**   5   _____

7. I am 65 years old or older.   **YES**   9   _____

TOTAL   _____

At-Risk Weight Chart

Height (in feet and inches without shoes)	Weight (in pounds without clothing)
4' 10"	129
4' 11"	133
5' 0"	138
5' 1"	143
5' 2"	147
5' 3"	152
5' 4"	157
5' 5"	162
5' 6"	167
5' 7"	172
5' 8"	177
5' 9"	182
5' 10"	188
5' 11"	193
6' 0"	199
6' 1"	204
6' 2"	210
6' 3"	216
6' 4"	221

Scoring:

10 or more points. You are at high risk for having diabetes. Only your health care provider can check to see if you have diabetes. See yours soon and find out for sure.

3 to 9 points. You are probably at low risk for having diabetes now. But don't just forget about it. Keep your risk low by losing weight if you are overweight, being active most days, and eating low fat meals that are high in fruits and vegetables and whole grain foods.

Reprinted with permission of the American Diabetes Association. **American Diabetes Association.**

A SERIOUS POINT

Carol could feel herself getting dizzy again as she stood up from her favorite chair. Probably she just shouldn't watch those reruns of *Seinfeld* back-to-back like that, she thought.

But what Carol could not feel was the 4-inch nail travel through her right foot so that its bloodied point now peeked through above her toes. Not until Carol went to take another step toward the kitchen and noticed a board sticking to her foot like an oversized flip-flop, in fact, did she have a clue anything was wrong. The nail had been projecting from a small plank that had come loose from the underside of Carol's recliner, and with no small help from her 260 pounds it had pierced through both the arch and instep of her foot.

Yet she "never felt a thing," Carol had to tell the emergency room doctor as he pried the plank free. For weeks her feet had been "pretty much totally numb," she had to confess, and lately she had begun to experience a similar loss of feeling in her hands. A quick blood test told why. Carol had diabetes, and it had begun to destroy the nerves in her hands and feet.

But the point of Carol's mishap, of course, is about more than just the nail. It's about how people who delay being diagnosed for diabetes invite so many complications that could be avoided with early detection. Carol's doctor told her that her case of diabetes probably had been festering for 10 to 15 years.

MOUNTAINS FROM MOLEHILLS

"Sure, it's frustrating," says past president of the American Diabetes Association (ADA), Gerald Bernstein, M.D., now a senior endocrinologist at Beth Israel Medical Center in New York. "Treatment can do so much for this disease, and especially if it's caught early. But people are waiting until they have symptoms, often serious symptoms, before getting help, and by then it can be too late to do much about them. What Dr. Bernstein is saying is that diabetes can be a very nasty disease—but it doesn't have to be. "And that's the real tragedy of this illness," he says. "So much of the disability and hardship diabetes causes could be prevented if more people would simply get themselves diagnosed in time."

Much of the hope we're justified in holding out for treating diabetes, in other words, lies not just in the hands of the doctors and research scientists dedicated to defeating the disease, but to "us," its potential victims. Yes, there are promising new treatments for diabetes, and even more on the horizon that could be available within just a few years. "But people need to avail themselves of treatment while they're still healthy enough to treat," Dr. Bernstein says. "Every day they wait, they give up a little bit more of themselves to this disease, and reduce their chances of being able to control it once treatment begins."

> *So much of the disability and hardship diabetes causes could be prevented if more people would simply get themselves diagnosed in time.*
>
> —GERALD BERNSTEIN, M.D.

High blood sugar levels in people with type 2 diabetes, for example, can begin to harm the pancreas—the very organ that produces the insulin needed to control high blood sugar in the first place. Similar types of vicious cycles can begin within the liver and kidneys, thus further compromising functions needed to keep diabetes under control. The disease, as a result, can begin to progress in an exponential fashion, with a little damage today leading to even more damage tomorrow. "It's a downward spiral that can be very difficult to stop, which points to the importance of not letting it begin in the first place," Dr. Bernstein says.

Today's molehill can becomes tomorrow's mountain, in other words, until diabetes can become all but impossible to surmount. The heart attacks, strokes, blindness, limb amputations, kidney disease, and sexual dysfunction in men and women alike, often occur because people go years, and sometimes even decades, before being diagnosed. "Yet the truth is that if people with diabetes would even come close to managing their conditions properly, they could live normal lives," Dr. Bernstein says. "And by that I mean to age 90 or even beyond."

NO HELP FROM HUMAN NATURE

But the key, of course, is being diagnosed in the first place, and making the tragedy of the disease all the more profound is how easy this diagnosis is to make. As you'll be seeing shortly, diabetes can be detected with just a simple blood test, a procedure that can be done by a family doctor or nurse in less time than it takes to order take-out at a fast-food restaurant.

A few minutes of testing to avoid a lifetime of woe—it should be a "no-brainer," right? The fact that diabetes, by some estimates, is our third leading cause of death by disease, suggests maybe not. For every case of diabetes that does get diagnosed, another case does *not*, the experts say, and for reasons that may have as much to do with human nature as the nature of the disease.

> *Diabetes can be detected with just a simple blood test, a procedure that can be done by a family doctor or nurse in less time than it takes to order take-out at a fast-food restaurant.*

"With type 2 diabetes, especially, symptoms can be subtle and develop slowly, so they tend to be ignored," Dr. Bernstein says. "Then, when symptoms do become obvious, they tend to be denied because diabetes has a reputation in many peoples' minds of being so difficult to treat. What people need to realize, however, is that compared to living with the complications of diabetes, living with treatment is a breeze."

As an example of the kind of denial Dr. Bernstein is talking about, consider another true story showing just how "convenient" it can be for diabetes to be overlooked. This story turns out with a happier ending than Carol's, as you'll see, but the point Dave's story makes is the same. Because diabetes can be like a volcano, showing little evidence of what trouble may be brewing below until it's too late, it can be very risky to wait until diabetes "erupts" before seeking help.

A CLOSE CALL

For more than a year, Dave had been telling himself it was just the side effects of his blood pressure medication—the thirst, the frequent trips to the bathroom, the occasional dizzy spells, and bouts of fatigue. Then one day Dave saw a program on public television about diabetes that included a list of the most common symptoms and, sure enough, he had to say yes to having 8 out of 10. But still Dave wasn't ready to put two and two together. He was too young to have diabetes, after all—only 43—and there was no history of the disease in his family. Besides, the idea of having to make major changes in his diet, and possibly even giving himself daily injections of insulin, seemed like a fate worse than the disease. He decided he'd just wait awhile and let nature take its course.

And a short course it was. While driving home from work about a week later, Dave nearly blacked out at the wheel, swerving dangerously into the opposing lane before regaining control. "It was a close call," he says, "and it really scared the daylights out of me because I had never experienced anything like it. I had this unbelievable thirst, too, and pains in my stomach, so I pulled over at the nearest pharmacy for help. I guess I

> *What people need to realize is that compared to living with the complications of diabetes, living with treatment is a breeze.*

must have looked pretty bad, too, because even before the guy at the counter asked if he could help me, he told me how terrible I looked."

And with that, Dave's denial broke down. "At first I tried to joke that I felt even worse than I looked, but the pharmacist wasn't laughing, and I guess that's when it hit me that maybe this diabetes thing was for real—and serious. So I told him what had happened and then asked if he thought it might be because of diabetes."

"That is very possible," the pharmacist said, offering Dave water and asking him to sit down while he did a quick test. Making due with a finger-pricking device (usually used for monitoring rather than diagnosing diabetes), the pharmacist found that Dave certainly was not crying wolf: At over 600 milligrams/deciliter, his glucose level was approximately six times higher than normal—an emergency situation. "The number 600 didn't mean anything to me," Dave recalls, "but 911 sure did."

The pharmacist was on the phone in a flash, calling for a police cruiser to rush Dave to the nearest hospital, and making Dave drink all the water he could to help his sugar-laden blood become more dilute. Once at the hospital, Dave was given a medication to help lower his glucose level further, followed by a blood test to see what might have caused such a massive glucose surge. Another test would be needed to confirm the diagnosis, he was told, but for the time being, it looked pretty certain: Dave appeared to have himself a whopping case of type 2 diabetes, a condition that probably had been in the making for several years.

When Dave asked why he had nearly blacked out, he was told he had a very serious condition known as *hypersomolar-nonketotic coma* whereby the body becomes so dehydrated trying to rid itself of glucose that not enough fluid remains even for the proper functioning of the brain. Had Dave not pulled into that pharmacy for help when he did, he very well could have lost consciousness and died.

WHY "WAIT AND SEE" DOESN'T WORK

Not all cases of diabetes make themselves known with the high-level drama of Dave's, of course, but they can be just as dangerous, nonetheless. Dave was lucky that his highway mishap was not more serious and lucky, too, that it drew attention to his condition before it had time to do more harm to his body. Rarely, however, is type 2 diabetes so helpful in making itself known. Unlike type 1 diabetes, which can develop quickly, the onset of type 2 usually is very slow, giving its sufferers little warning until considerable damage has been done.

"I guess I was just hoping my symptoms would go way," Dave now says, "but I learned pretty quickly from my doctor that's not the way diabetes works."

Not by a long shot. "The wait-and-see attitude can be a real problem with diabetes," says Corina Graziani, M.D., the diabetes educator from Thomas Jefferson University Hospital we met in chapter 1. "Diabetes never gets better if left untreated," she says. "It always, in fact, will get worse."

> *Diabetes never gets better if left untreated. It always, in fact, will get worse.*
>
> —CORINA GRAZIANI, M.D.

A quick reminder of what causes diabetes in the first place should explain why. Diabetes is caused by high levels of sugar in the blood that, over time, can begin to compromise the functioning of the very organs that play a role in keeping glucose levels under control. Diabetes can begin to damage the liver, which is involved in blood sugar control, for example, and even the pancreas, whose job it is to produce glucose-taming insulin in the first place. The disease can begin to gather momentum from the very complications it causes, in other words, creating a vicious cycle indeed.

TEST EARLY, ESPECIALLY IF OVERWEIGHT

This is why it's always best to be tested for diabetes even if there's the slightest suspicion it may exist, the experts agree. "There is no question that the sooner the disease is caught, the sooner it can be treated and the less damage it can do," Dr. Bernstein says.

Those are words we all might want to tape to our refrigerator doors, especially if we're opening those doors often. Being overweight is without a doubt the number one preventable risk factor for type 2 diabetes, even in people, as Dave thought, "too young" to have the disease. "That's been the real eye-opener for diabetes researchers in recent years," Dr. Bernstein says.

Type 2 diabetes is now so prevalent in overweight people in their 20s and even teens, in fact, that the American Diabetes Association no longer designates the illness as an "adult-onset" disease. The term "obesity-onset" might be more accurate, and for reasons not hard to understand. Fat cells simply aren't as receptive to insulin as muscle cells, so the more fat in relation to muscle that you have, the more insulin-resistant and hence more susceptible to type 2 diabetes you're going to be. "Other problems associated with obesity such as high blood pressure and high blood fats also can increase diabetes risks," Dr. Bernstein says, "so it's clear that the overweight, even while still relatively young, need to be the most vigilant of all against this disease."

> *Type 2 diabetes is now so prevalent in overweight people in their 20s and even teens that the American Diabetes Association no longer designates the illness as an "adult-onset" disease.*

Dave, as an example, started to gain weight in his 20s when his job in sales demanded little more than marathon drives in his car, which he helped make tolerable by snacking on candy bars and unwinding at night by drinking four or five beers in front of the TV. It wasn't long before his once athletic 180 pounds ballooned to 260 and his blood pressure skyrocketed, too. Even without a family history of the disease, and without a single gray hair, Dave had become an all-too-likely candidate for what he had considered an "old person's" disease.

Dave's misconception is a common one, and it's unfortunate that it is, Dr. Bernstein says, because it prevents many people from getting treatment when it could do the most good. "It's always worthwhile and important to treat diabetes at any stage, of course, but the chances for success are far greater when treatment begins before complications have had a chance to occur."

That said, Dr. Bernstein recommends that age be no obstacle in being tested. Anyone—regardless of age—should have a blood test for diabetes, he says, if any of the following conditions apply:

- You are 20 percent or more overweight.

- You have a history of diabetes in your family.

- You are of African American, Hispanic, Asian, Pacific Island, or Native American decent.

- You have high blood pressure or elevated blood fats.

- You have had diabetes during a pregnancy (gestational diabetes) or have given birth to a baby weighing more than 9 pounds.

DIAGNOSIS: WHAT TO EXPECT

So what does being tested for diabetes involve?

Considering all the suffering it can avoid, amazingly little. Unlike other chronic diseases such as heart disease or cancer for which diagnosis may require tests that are time-consuming, invasive, expensive, or painful, testing for diabetes is a relative breeze. When our "denizen of denial" Dave, for example, was rushed to the hospital after his diabetes nearly caused him to crash his car, he was surprised at how fast and easy the diagnostic procedure turned out to be. "Is that all there is?" he asked the nurse after she had painlessly drawn several small samples of blood.

As explained shortly, there are different ways to test for diabetes, but they all have one thing in common: They measure what constitutes diabetes in the first place, which is abnormally high levels of glucose in the blood. Let's take a look now at the various tests themselves.

Random Plasma Glucose Test

This test, as its name implies, measures the amount of glucose in the blood at random, meaning at no special time with respect to when the person being tested has last eaten. A small sample of blood is drawn, usually from the forearm, and if glucose levels are found to be 200 milligrams/deciliter (specifically, milligrams of glucose per deciliter of blood) or higher, and other signs of diabetes such as fatigue, extreme thirst, and frequent urination also are present, diabetes usually will be diagnosed. (In a person without diabetes, by comparison, glucose levels rarely will exceed 140 milligrams/deciliter even after a feast.)

Fasting Plasma Glucose Test

This is a more definitive method of testing for diabetes because it eliminates the variable of glucose levels being affected by the process of digestion (as the random method of testing mentioned above does not). Blood is drawn after the patient has not eaten for a period of 8 to 10 hours, and if the amount of glucose in the blood is found to be 126 milligrams/deciliter or higher, diabetes will be suspected. To confirm the diagnosis, however, another test may be repeated on a subsequent day, and if it, too, yields glucose levels at or above the mark of 126 milligrams/deciliter, diabetes usually will be confirmed. (In people without diabetes, fasting blood sugar levels usually are under 110 milligrams/deciliter.)

The ADA currently recommends that everyone over the age of 45—regardless of risk factors normally associated with diabetes—should have a fasting plasma glucose (FPG) test at least every 3 years. If any risk factors are present, however, or any telltale symptoms occur (see "Classic Symptoms" beginning on page 53), the FPG should be taken regardless of age. And if results of the FPG are between 110 and 125, the test should be retaken at least yearly.

Glucose Challenge

This is a diabetes test given to pregnant women between the 24th and 28th week of pregnancy to test for gestational diabetes. The person being tested is given a drink containing glucose; then, about 2 hours later, blood is drawn to see how the drink has affected glucose levels in the blood. If the amount of glucose remaining in the blood is found to be 140 milligrams/deciliter or higher, gestational diabetes will be suspected but not confirmed until a subsequent fasting glucose test also produces positive results.

Glucose Tolerance Test

Often a person tested for diabetes will produce results that are considered borderline, in which case a procedure known as a *glucose tolerance test* may be called for. The patient is asked to eat a large amount of foods high in carbohydrates for 3 days prior to being tested. Then, having fasted since dinner the night before the test on day 4, the person is given a blood glucose test to establish a baseline. The patient then drinks a solution high in glucose, which is followed by subsequent blood tests done at regular intervals to see how the glucose in the drink is being handled.

Glycated Hemoglobin Testing

In addition to the tests above, which give readings of blood glucose levels at the time of the test only, another type of glucose monitoring has been developed that gives valuable information on the body's ability to regulate blood sugar levels over an extended period. The test works by measuring the amount of a substance in the blood called *glycated hemoglobin*, a variation of regular hemoglobin that forms when hemoglobin bonds to molecules of glucose. The more glucose that is present in the blood, the higher glycated hemoglobin levels will be, and since this process of glycation takes several weeks to occur, the test is able to assess the body's average glucose level over periods of as long as 2 to 3 months. This makes the test a valuable addition to the other types of tests, which give readings that reflect glucose levels for periods of perhaps only a few hours. For this reason, both types of tests should be given to produce the most accurate picture possible of how and when blood sugar levels may be deviating from the norm.

"Not Quite" Diabetes: Impaired Glucose Tolerance

Sometimes tests indicate a condition that does not constitute diabetes but is cause for concern, nonetheless. It's called *impaired glucose tolerance*, and it can lead to diabetes in many cases. Even if impaired glucose tolerance does not progress to diabetes, however, people with the condition can suffer from some of the same complications produced by "the real thing," and they're at increased risk for heart disease as well. For this reason, people with impaired glucose tolerance usually are advised to keep in close contact with their physicians and also to undertake the same lifestyle changes of weight control and regular exercise to keep their conditions from getting worse. In some cases, diligent management of impaired glucose tolerance can return blood sugar responses to normal, thus essentially stopping diabetes before it starts.

> *Even if impaired glucose tolerance does not progress to diabetes, people with the condition can suffer from some of the same complications produced by "the real thing."*

WHY GET TESTED FOR DIABETES?

As we saw in the cases of Carol and Dave, one of the most insidious aspects of diabetes is how easy its symptoms are to ignore. Not only do they usually develop slowly, but they often are easily attributed to something else. Fatigue or irritability, for example, is easy to blame on lack of sleep. Numbness or tingling in the feet might be attributed to "bad circulation" or poorly fitting shoes. Even something as alarming as episodes of blurred vision may be seen just as time for a new pair of glasses. (Our "master of denial" Dave went so far as to wonder at times whether his increased thirst might have had something to do with global warming.)

As we're finding excuses, however, diabetes is finding a foothold. As explained by the ADA's past president, Gerald Bernstein, M.D., "Having diabetes is like taking a cup of honey, putting your hand in it, and walking around the house touching all your belongings. Glucose hooks on to proteins in tissues, then that's attracted to other tissues with excess glucose. They bind to each other and eventually vessels just close up."

And that means vessels of all types—everywhere. The body's largest blood vessels begin to narrow, increasing risks for heart attacks and strokes as the stickiness of the blood encourages the buildup of fat particles and other debris on artery walls. Hit even harder are the body's smallest blood vessels (capillaries), which can clog up completely, causing tissue served by those vessels to die. Small ductways in the body's major organs also can begin to narrow and clog, creating very "sticky" situations, indeed, as these organs can gradually cease to function.

The message, in short, is don't feel it's just "all in your head" if you experience any of these symptoms and have any reason to suspect diabetes may be the cause. Contact your doctor, and discuss whether he or she feels a test for diabetes may be in order. "Many of our patients discover they have diabetes in this sort of backdoor fashion," says John Stringfield, M.D., a family practitioner and codirector of Waynesville Family Practice, in Waynesville, North Carolina. "They come in complaining of fatigue, or dizziness, or an infection, or any of the other telltale signs of diabetes, and a routine blood test shows they've got glucose levels through the roof."

Classic Symptoms

Keep in mind that by being diagnosed on the basis of having just one or a few of the following symptoms, you can begin treatment in time to reduce your chances of suffering from others. Common symptoms of diabetes include:

- **Lack of energy**. Because type 2 diabetes is caused by the inability of the body's cells to absorb glucose for the production of energy, it should come as no surprise that a lack of energy is often the result. The body is "out of gas" because it can't make use of the gas (glucose) it has.

- **Blurred vision**. As glucose accumulates in the blood, it also accumulates in the fluid of the eyes. This not only changes the way these fluids refract light, but the glucose absorbs water, which causes the outer lens of the eye to swell, thus distorting the shape of the lens and also the objects the lens tries to bring into focus.

- **Frequent urination and thirst**. The body responds to high levels of sugar in the blood by mobilizing body fluids in an attempt to thin the blood down. This results in frequent urination and consequently increased thirst to replace the fluids being lost.

- **Tingling, numbness, or pain in the hands or feet**. Diabetes can damage the body's nerves by causing glucose to infiltrate the cells that make up the coating that surrounds nerves for protection. This infiltration can cause the coating to swell, thus producing pain as pressure is exerted on the nerves inside. If nerves within the muscle are involved (called *sensory neuropathy*), tingling or numbness in the hands or feet may develop.

- **Dizzy spells**. Nerves controlling the expansion and contraction of the blood vessels can be harmed by diabetes, leading to dizzy spells caused by sudden drops in blood pressure, especially when standing up after periods of extended sitting.

- **Sexual dysfunction**. Because diabetes can adversely affect both nerve function and blood flow to and within the sex organs—in both sexes—the disease can produce erectile failure in men and vaginal dryness in women.

- **Digestive problems**. These can include constipation, diarrhea, nausea, vomiting, and abdominal pain, which may result when diabetes damages nerve function responsible for the muscular contractions of the intestines and stomach. A condition known as *gastroparesis* may develop, for example, which results when the stomach is unable to empty itself properly after meals.

- **Slow healing wounds or frequent infections**. By suppressing the immune system, diabetes increases risks not just for local infections of all types—bladder and vaginal, included—but also full-body infections such as colds and flu. Excess glucose in the blood interferes with the germ-fighting activity of white blood cells as it also gives bacteria and other pathogens food (sugar) to feed on.

- **Moodiness**. Because diabetes can cause so many major changes in the body, it should come as no surprise that it can cause changes in mood as well. People with diabetes frequently complain of feeling irritable and depressed, especially when their glucose levels are not being well controlled.

THE FOUR CORNERSTONES OF TREATMENT

And what if test results give your doctor cause for concern?

Let no question go unasked. Ask your doctor to explain in as much detail as possible what your tests show. Do they indicate how advanced your condition might be? Might you already have begun to develop any complications from your condition that will need treatment, and might you be at risk for developing others?

When Dave was first diagnosed with type 2 diabetes, for example, he was told he was lucky to have come for help when he did. No, his condition did not appear to have done any discernible damage yet, but it was at a stage where it was about to.

> *Let no question go unasked. Ask your doctor to explain in as much detail as possible what your tests show.*

Right away, therefore, the emergency room doctor who made Dave's preliminary diagnosis referred Dave to a diabetes expert, an endocrinologist who would be overseeing additional tests to find out more about Dave's condition. The endocrinologist would also be acting as the leader of a "team" of other experts responsible for Dave's treatment. At their first meeting, the endocrinologist explained to Dave what would be the four most important aspects of his treatment program. (We'll be looking at each of these in more detail in subsequent chapters, but they're offered here to help you begin thinking in the right directions.)

1. Diet

Yes, Dave would definitely need to make some changes here. The morning donut would have to go, replaced by a more nutritious breakfast lower in saturated fat and higher in dietary fiber and protein. Lunch also would have to be revised to reduce fat and increase fiber content, and his evening meal would need to be trimmed of its fat and bulked up in the fiber department, too. Dave also was going to have to start eating on a more regular schedule, not the feast-or-famine style he'd been used to. The goal of this diet, his doctor explained, was threefold: It was to help Dave lose weight, to lower the amount of fat (cholesterol and triglycerides) in his blood, and also to keep his blood sugar levels as stable as possible. The weight loss, his doctor went on to explain, would control Dave's blood pressure in addition to making his body be more sensitive to the limited amounts of insulin his pancreas was still managing to produce. The reduced fat intake would lower his blood fats and hence his risks of heart disease and stroke, and by helping normalize his glucose levels through diet, Dave would be minimizing his need for glucose-controlling medication.

But could such a diet be satisfying? That would be up to him and his wife to determine, his doctor said, offering that many excellent cookbooks were available to help them.

2. Exercise

Dave had played three sports in high school, so he knew what it meant to be in shape, but he did have to admit that he'd let himself go in recent years. But was it going to have to be wind sprints and push-ups all over again? Hardly, his doctor assured him. The purpose of exercise wasn't to get Dave on the cover of a muscle magazine, but simply to get his muscle cells more active so they could help use up the extra glucose that was accumulating in his blood. A half-hour walk most days of the week would probably be enough. That amount of exercise not only would help stabilize Dave's blood sugar but also would help him lose weight and lower his blood pressure. Yet another bonus would be the tendency of exercise to raise HDLs (high-density lipoproteins)—blood particles that help carry cholesterol in the blood off to the liver for disposal before it can increase the risk of heart disease by accumulating on artery walls. There would be a positive emotional component Dave would get from exercise, too, which would be important in helping him deal with the mental stress of his disease.

3. Medication

Dave's doctor told him he'd be starting him on two oral medications, in pill form. One (of a class of drugs called *sulfonylureas*) would help stimulate Dave's pancreas to produce more insulin, while the other (belonging to a group known as *biguanides*) would help his cells be more insulin-sensitive while also curbing the amount of glucose released by his liver. In conjunction with the dietary and exercise changes Dave would be making, his doctor felt these oral medications would be enough. If not, insulin injections might be called for, but he said they'd cross that bridge if they got to it. It would largely be up to Dave, and the effort he was willing to invest, to see whether that recourse would be needed.

4. Monitoring

Last but not least, Dave would need to keep track of his blood sugar levels using a small finger-pricking device at regular intervals throughout the day. His doctor advised once before breakfast and again before his evening meal until his appropriate medication levels could be determined. Once Dave had his treatment program well in place, fewer testings might be possible, but his doctor warned Dave of the dangers of assuming all is well just because Dave might not be experiencing any adverse symptoms. His blood sugar could be dangerously high, and he still might not feel noticeably different. His monitoring always would be able to tell Dave "the truth," so it was a trusty tool he should not take lightly.

ASSEMBLING A "DREAM TEAM" OF HEALTH EXPERTS

While it's true that most primary care physicians (family doctors) are able to diagnose diabetes by administering one or more of the tests mentioned earlier, treatment of the disease is best entrusted to a health care team that specializes in the illness. As with many other serious health problems, even the best general practitioner may not be aware of all the concerns that need to be addressed in treating this very complex and individual disease. No two cases of diabetes are exactly alike, so no two treatment programs will be exactly alike. The degree of success any treatment program is likely to have, in fact, will depend on the degree to which it is customized to accommodate the patient's particular condition, lifestyle, temperament, and emotional as well as family and workplace concerns.

> *No two cases of diabetes are exactly alike, so no two treatment programs will be exactly alike.*

Many medical centers and hospitals offer specially trained diabetes treatment teams, already assembled, that can help the person with diabetes manage his or her disease as effectively as medically possible. If not, such a team may need to be created with the help of the patient's family doctor. In either case, the health care team should include the following experts to assure that all aspects of this complex disease are adequately addressed:

- **Diabetologist.** A physician specially trained in diabetes management who often will be board-certified in endocrinology.

- **Nurse educator.** A nurse who specializes in the management of diabetes and usually will be credentialed as a certified diabetes educator (CDE).

- **Registered dietician.** A dietician whose training has been specific to the nutritional needs of people with diabetes, including the most effective and healthful ways to help patients lose weight without having to sacrifice sound nutrition or good taste. Often a registered dietician is also a CDE.

- **Exercise physiologist.** An expert trained to help people with diabetes get the exercise they need to make their bodies more responsive to insulin and also to lose weight.

- **Mental health specialist.** A psychiatrist, psychologist, or social worker whose role is a crucial one: helping the diabetic patient and his or her family deal with the emotional and social impacts of the disease.

In addition to benefiting from the expert assistance of a team of such specialists, many people with diabetes can gain valuable insights by attending diabetes support groups or attending educational programs offered at hospitals or medical centers specializing in treatment of the disease.

Specialists for Special Concerns

The specialists just mentioned generally are considered the core members of a diabetic health care team, but there may be a need to consult one or more of the following experts if more specific complications develop.

Ophthalmologist

Because diabetes can damage the tiny blood vessels of the eyes, it's important for patients to have their eyes checked regularly. Patients over the age of 30 should have a thorough eye exam at the time of diagnosis and then yearly after that, while patients between ages 12 and 30 should have yearly exams if they've had diabetes for at least 5 years. Patients also should be sure to contact their ophthalmologist as soon as any changes in their vision occurs. This is critical because the earlier eye problems are discovered the more successfully they can be treated. Here are some pertinent questions patients should ask an ophthalmologist before enlisting his or her services:

- Is the ophthalmologist experienced in treating diabetic patients?
- Does the ophthalmologist perform eye surgery?
- Is the ophthalmologist an expert in treating problems of the retina?
- Will the ophthalmologist submit regular reports and keep in touch with the patient's primary care physician?

Podiatrist

Proper care of the feet is especially important for people with diabetes because the disease can inhibit blood flow and also disrupt normal nerve function in the extremities. Diabetes also can make infection more likely in the feet, turning what might seem like a minor sore or callus into a potentially serious problem very quickly. Patients should ask their primary care physician for the name of a podiatrist or check with their local ADA chapter or affiliate. In addition to taking special foot care precautions on their own (see below), patients should see their podiatrists immediately if any of the following problems occurs:

- An open sore
- Any infection of a cut or blister
- A toe that becomes red or tender, possibly indicating an in-grown toenail
- Any change in feeling, such as pain, numbness, burning, or tingling
- Any puncture wound

Nephrologist

Because diabetes sometimes can begin to damage the kidneys, especially if not well controlled or if the patient also has high blood pressure, some patients may need to consult a doctor specializing in kidney problems known as a *nephrologist*. It usually takes many years for kidney disease to occur because the kidneys are an especially resilient organ, but if it does, a low-salt diet and special type of blood pressure medication may be prescribed. If the damage is more advanced, a low-protein diet also may be recommended, and in the most severe cases, dialysis (a process that does the kidneys' job of filtering toxins from the blood artificially) or even a kidney transplant may be required.

FINDING DR. RIGHT

Because diabetes is best managed when the treatment program matches the individual needs of the patient as closely as possible, it should come as no surprise that the same compatibility should exist between the patient and the doctor in charge of overseeing that program. This doctor, usually an *endocrinologist*, will be the person to whom most of the patient's concerns will initially be addressed, so a good personal relationship should prevail, as well as a strong feeling of confidence that the doctor has the right qualifications for the job.

That said, here are some key questions the ADA recommends that patients ask a prospective doctor in a personal interview before entrusting themselves to his or her care:

- Where has the doctor attended medical school?
- Is the doctor board-certified in either endocrinology or internal medicine?
- Is the doctor a member of the American Diabetes Association, the Endocrine Society, or the American College of Physicians?
- What percentage of the doctor's patients are being treating for diabetes (the higher, the better)?
- Will the doctor accept the appropriate insurance plan?
- How frequently will appointments be required?

Too Civilized for Our Own Good?

To understand the proliferation of diabetes in the modern world, former American Diabetes president Gerald Bernstein, M.D., says it can be helpful to look back a few hundred thousand years to the conditions under which we evolved. "There wasn't a fast-food restaurant on every corner, that's for sure."

We were hunter-gatherers, Dr. Bernstein says, which meant we pretty much kept moving all day long and probably were getting just enough calories to survive. Compare that to today when so many of us sit all day long at our jobs, then just pop some high-calorie feast into a microwave oven or phone for a pepperoni pizza for dinner.

For thousands of years our bodies were used to running hard, in other words, and a lot of the time on near "empty." But now we're being allowed to just sit, usually with "full tanks." All this has happened in a span of less than a hundred years, moreover, a mere drop

- Who covers for the doctor on days off, and what are their credentials?
- What procedures should be followed in the event of an emergency and what conditions constitute an emergency?
- Does the doctor work in conjunction with other health care professionals, thus offering the benefits of a well-coordinated team approach?

It's important that these questions are answered satisfactorily not just in substance but also in style. Is the doctor the type of person who genuinely seems to care and with whom the patient can feel comfortable? If not, other candidates should be considered through referral from the local hospital or community health organization, local chapter of the ADA, or the patient's primary care physician.

in the bucket given the tens of thousands of years it took for our bodies to evolve under those much harsher conditions.

"Our metabolisms, you might say, have been slow to catch up," Dr. Bernstein says. Today's land of plenty—with no physical effort required to enjoy it—has thrown our bodies something of a biochemical curve ball.

But if our world today is so "unnatural," why should some of us get diabetes and not others?

We may need to blame a certain "thrifty gene," Dr. Bernstein says, the one passed along by our prehistoric ancestors who were better able to store calories as fat rather than burn them quickly for energy. "These were our predecessors who were the most likely to survive famines and hence pass the thrifty gene along," Dr. Bernstein points out.

It's an irony, certainly. Yesterday's blessing is today's curse. The propensity for becoming obese—once a key to health—is now a leading cause of disease.

GETTING EDUCATED

Because diabetes is such a complex disease that can develop in so many different ways, it's important for every patient to become as knowledgeable about his or her particular condition as possible. This book will help, of course, but additional information can be obtained by attending diabetes education programs. Contact the local chapter of the ADA for information on the availability of such a program near you.

It's also important for patients to be able to talk as openly as possible with their health care providers. This is sometimes difficult because doctors can be reluctant to spend much of their valuable time in explaining treatment procedures. Even when they are willing, moreover, the terms they use can be so technical they can be difficult to understand. But for diabetes to be treated successfully, there must be good communication between doctor and patient, so here are some tips on making that communication as valuable as possible:

- Don't be afraid to express your feelings and concerns about all aspects of your treatment.
- Ask questions if the discussion begins to get too scientific, and there are things you don't understand.
- Try not to be shy about asking sensitive questions that may relate to personal or sexual matters.
- Feel free to express any financial concerns.
- Don't be afraid to consult a different doctor if you feel a communication barrier with your current one.

A CHANCE FOR A LIFETIME

Has this chapter made an impression on you? Hopefully it has, because the importance of being diagnosed early for diabetes can't be stressed enough. Much like running a car when its engine is low on oil can do progressively more damage with every passing mile, allowing diabetes to go untreated can do increasingly more harm to the body with every passing day—and it's damage that can't be repaired.

Besides, once treatment begins, you're likely to feel better, and not just in the long run, but right away. You're likely to notice more energy, for example, as your body once again will be able to use glucose for fuel, and you may experience less moodiness as your blood sugar becomes more stabilized. If constant thirst and frequent urination have been problems, expect to say good-bye to these, too. You may even be able to say farewell to some hard-to-lose pounds if your diagnosis reveals that your body has been accumulating too much fat-storing insulin.

Treatment can help you live not just longer, in other words, but considerably better, too. It's a chance of a lifetime—because it's a chance *for* a lifetime—not to be missed.

CHAPTER 3

The Miracles of Medical Treatment

❧

D ON'T TELL ME about diabetes. I watched my grandfather, my mother, and an uncle die of the disease, and nothing they did seemed to make any difference. Why should I torture myself if it's going to be the same way with me?"

That line of thinking, unfortunately, has done more to hinder progress against diabetes than any ice cream cone or extra serving of mashed potatoes. People see what devastation the disease may have caused loved ones in the past, assume that's the way it will be for them in the future, and in the process ignore what they *could* be doing for themselves in the present.

But looking backward, of course, is not the way to make progress in any endeavor, especially not medical science. Medical science responds to the needs of today for the assurance of a better tomorrow, and the needs demanded by diabetes have been considerable, to say the least. Incidence of the disease has tripled since 1960 alone, and when a disease inflicts as much hardship as diabetes, it's going to get the attention of some of the very best scientific minds in the world. Diabetes has, and the attention has paid off.

Researchers have never known as much about diabetes—its causes, how to prevent it, and how to limit its devastating effects—as they do today. That boast comes from the American Diabetes Association, and it's not an idle one. Diabetes was a virtual death sentence as recently as 80 years ago, but today people with the disease can live long, healthy, and normal lives. The understanding and treatment of diabetes comprise one of modern medicine's greatest feats.

And the best may be still to come. Currently there are no cures for diabetes, only the highly effective treatments we'll be learning about in this chapter, but it's nice to know we can remain hopeful that such cures will come. As we'll be seeing in chapter 8, scientists currently are pursuing new breakthroughs that could lead to cures for both type 1 and type 2 diabetes in the relatively near future, ADA officials say.

But we can't count those eggs yet, of course, so let's take a look at what breakthroughs have been hatched in the way of treatment for this once untreatable disease. First we'll look at the impressive new array of oral medications now available for helping keep type 2 diabetes under control. Then we'll examine new developments that have made it easier to use the old granddad of diabetes treatments, insulin, which remains the mainstay of treatment for type 1 diabetes but also is needed by as many as 40 percent of people with type 2. Then, in chapter 4, we'll look at what may be the most critical of all aspects of successful treatment—the best ways to monitor glucose levels so that the new medications can be used with optimal effect.

It's a lot to cover, fortunately—proof of just how hard diabetes researchers have been working so that we *can* make a difference against this disease, after all.

NO TWO CASES OF TYPE 2 ARE ALIKE

To understand the latest medicines for treating type 2 diabetes, it's important to remember just how different each case of the disease can be. Unlike type 1 diabetes that is relatively "simple" in that high glucose levels result from the pancreas being unable to produce any appreciable insulin at all, type 2 is more complex because it can cause high glucose levels for one or more of the following reasons:

- The pancreas may not be producing insulin in sufficient quantity.

- The pancreas may not be producing insulin that's of a sufficient quality.

- The body's cells may have lost their ability to respond to insulin even if the pancreas is producing insulin as it should.

- The liver may be adding insult to injury by releasing glucose of its own into a bloodstream burdened with too much glucose as it is. (See the sidebar "The Role the Liver Plays.")

> *Researchers have never known as much about diabetes— its causes, how to prevent it, and how to limit its devastating effects— as they do today.*

The challenge in treating type 2 diabetes, therefore, becomes one of determining which of these possible causes—or combination of causes— is exerting the greatest influence so that the right combination of dietary advice, exercise recommendations, and medications, if necessary, can be used to best normalize glucose levels.

We'll be looking at dietary and exercise therapies in chapter 6, so our focus here will be on the "meds," as they're now often called. No, none of these medications is able to cure diabetes, but they can help stop the disease from doing harm, saving millions of lives and livelihoods in the process.

MEDICATIONS FOR TYPE 2 DIABETES

When Pat learned she had diabetes at age 51, her first thought was a near mortal one. "There's simply no way I'll ever be able to give myself injections of insulin," she said. "I think I'd die just trying."

The Role the Liver Plays (It Can Be a "Spoiler")

We tend to think of type 2 diabetes as a problem that exists primarily between the pancreas and the body's cells, as the two fail to coordinate in making proper use of insulin for the purpose of deriving energy from glucose. This scenario, however, neglects a "third party"—namely, the liver—which also can play a critical role in the onset and progression of this disease. Normally the liver's job is to release glucose into the bloodstream when supplies from the food we eat run low—during the night as we're sleeping, for example, or in response to extreme physical exertion that can cause glucose supplies in the blood to run low. The liver does this job based on the amount of insulin in the blood: When insulin levels are high, it correctly assumes that high glucose levels must be the reason, so it's careful not to add any more glucose to the mix.

Not so in some cases of type 2 diabetes. For reasons not fully understood, the liver, in a sense, becomes "blind" to high insulin levels. This blindness by the liver wouldn't be a problem if the organ would recognize its shortcoming and sit tight, but it doesn't. Not only does the liver fail to see that insulin levels are rising; it fails to see any insulin at all, and it makes the very serious error of assuming

Scientists may well have understood this pervasive fear of needles when they set out to create today's current lineup of medications for type 2 diabetes—all can be taken in pill form. Unlike insulin that must be injected because it's a naturally occurring protein easily broken down by the process of digestion, diabetes pills are synthetically derived chemical compounds that, in fact, rely on digestion for getting into the bloodstream by way of the stomach and small intestine.

Currently many different types and brands of diabetes drugs are being used in the United States, but most fall into one of three basic categories depending on their primary mode of action:

this to mean there's not enough glucose in the blood for insulin to be working on. Hoping to save the day, the liver begins releasing its own glucose into the blood, and whammo—suddenly there's more glucose in the blood than ever.

Not only does this raise glucose levels to even more toxic levels, of course, but it signals the pancreas to step up its output of insulin in hopes of correcting the situation, the result now being two problems rather than just one—high insulin levels and high glucose levels combined. This spells trouble, because in addition to helping cells use glucose, insulin helps cells store fat, so greater amounts mean greater fat storage, and that's the last thing a type 2 diabetic needs. More insulin means greater chances for weight gain, which in most people with type 2 diabetes has been a major factor in their becoming insulin-resistant—and thus diabetic—in the first place.

It can become a vicious cycle as weight gain produces more insulin resistance, which makes the pancreas put out more insulin, which produces more weight gain and hence more insulin resistance. This is why weight loss and also exercise can be so helpful in treating type 2 diabetes: They can help correct the insulin resistance that gives this vicious cycle its start.

1. Stimulating the pancreas to increase its insulin output.

2. Making the body's cells more sensitive to insulin so the cells can increase their glucose uptake.

3. Preventing or slowing the digestion of starches and other sugars in the diet so that less glucose enters the bloodstream in the first place.

There's a certain amount of crossover between categories—meaning some medications perform more than just one of these three basic glucose-controlling functions—but more on that as we give the medications a closer look.

The point needs to be made here that whatever medication or combination of medications your doctor may determine is best for you, it will be a regimen custom-tailored to fit your particular needs.

> *Scientists may well have understood the pervasive fear of needles when they set out to create today's current lineup of medications for type 2 diabetes—all can be taken in pill form.*

There is no "one-size-fits-all" approach to prescribing drugs for type 2 diabetes, in other words. The new lineup of medications allows doctors a great deal of flexibility in creating a treatment program that is the best possible match for each individual patient—very important, indeed, given just how "individual" each case of type 2 diabetes can be. Often this means that several medications will be prescribed at the same time—one to induce more insulin output, for example, another to spur greater insulin sensitivity, and possibly even a third type to reduce the amount of glucose that the body's insulin supplies need to deal with in the first place.

The success that can be achieved by the use of several medications at once can be truly remarkable, but as Dr. Bernstein makes very clear, contributing lifestyle factors also must be addressed. "These type 2 medications mustn't be thought of as a substitute for healthful eating and exercise," he says. "Anyone who relies on medications alone to keep blood sugar under control is going to be very disappointed. The drugs must be used as part of a unified effort in which diet and exercise play an equally important role."

Alan L. Rubin, M.D., a member of the American Diabetes Association and author of the book *Diabetes for Dummies*, who's been treating diabetes for more than 25 years, agrees. "No drug should be taken as a convenient way of avoiding the basic diet and exercise that is the key to diabetic control."

Keep that well in mind as we look at what these new drugs can do. The results that can be expected of them will depend on the degree to which they are complemented by an antidiabetes lifestyle.

Drugs That Boost Insulin Output

Sulfonylureas comprise a class of medications discovered accidentally during World War II when doctors noticed that soldiers given antibacterial drugs containing sulfur experienced symptoms of low blood sugar. Eureka! Scientists quickly got to work on perfecting these drugs for the expressed purpose of treating diabetes, and by the 1950s, several medications were successfully being used, many of which remain in use today. These drugs work primarily by stimulating insulin output from the pancreas, and although they're the oldest medications for treating type 2 diabetes, they're still among the most widely prescribed, often in conjunction with one or more additional medications for a more complete treatment program.

> *The new lineup of medications allows doctors a great deal of flexibility in creating a treatment program that is the best possible match for each individual patient—very important, indeed, given just how individual each case of type 2 diabetes can be.*

The sulfonylureas currently available in the United States are listed here. The first four belong to a class known as the "first generation" of these drugs, while the last three are updated versions known as the "second generation." All have similar effects on blood sugar, but they can differ in how often they should be taken, their possible side effects, and their interactions with other medications. (If you have any questions about dosage instructions, drug interactions, or side effects, be sure to check with your doctor. These medications also may cause adverse reactions in people allergic to drugs in the "sulfa" family, so this matter should be discussed with your doctor as well.) It should be noted, too, that as widely prescribed as these sulfa-based drugs are, and as effective as they can be, they all have the common drawback of becoming less effective with prolonged use.

First-Generation Sulfonylureas

The fact that some of these medications have been in use for decades can be considered a testimony to their worth:

- **Tolbutamide (brand name Orinase)**. This is the fastest-acting of the sulfonylureas, taking effect within an hour but lasting for only about 10 hours. Usually it's taken three times daily, before meals, but for some people one or two doses daily is enough. It comes in 250- and 500-milligram strengths with the maximum dose put at 3 grams (six 500-milligram pills) daily.

- **Acetohexamide (Dymelor)**. This drug also works quickly, usually within about an hour, and remains active for approximately 12 hours. It comes in 250- and 500-milligram doses, which usually are taken once or twice a day. The maximum dose is 1.5 grams, or three 500-milligram tablets daily. Because by-products created by this medication need to be excreted in the urine, it is not a good choice for people suffering from kidney problems.

- **Tolazamide (Tolinase)**. This medication is absorbed more slowly than other sulfonylureas—usually not for 4 hours or more—but a single dose can last for up to 20 hours. It comes in strengths of 100, 250, and 500 milligrams, with 1,000 milligrams being the maximum to be taken in any one day. Like acetohexamide, however, it's not advised for people suffering from kidney disease.

- **Chlorpropamide (Diabinase, Glucamide)**. This is the longest-lasting of the first generation sulfonylureas—remaining active for up to 24 hours—but with this longevity can come a price: Chlorpropamide can cause blood sugar levels to fall too low in some patients, sometimes to a point where glucose must be given intravenously. The drug also can cause water retention, and facial flushing can result if it's used in conjunction with alcohol. The medication comes in 100- and 250-milligram strengths, with 750 milligrams not to be exceeded daily.

Second-Generation Sulfonylureas

Although the first generation sulfonylureas are still used, and are appropriate for some patients in whom stronger medications might drive glucose levels too low, they largely have been replaced by this group of more potent newcomers:

- **Glyburide (Micronase, Diabeta, Glynase).** This medication comes in 1.25-, 2.5-, and 5-milligram strengths, and while it may cause low blood sugar in some cases—especially if taken with other medications such as aspirin that bind to proteins in the bloodstream—chances of other side effects generally are very low.

- **Glipizide (Glucotrol, Glucotrol XL).** To be taken 30 minutes before meals, glipizide comes in 5- and 10-milligram doses and is similar to glyburide but slightly less potent, making it a good choice for the elderly. Glucotrol XL, which also comes in 5- and 10-milligram strengths, is an extended-release form of glipizide that usually needs to be taken only once a day.

- **Glimepiride (Amaryl).** This is another long-acting sulfonylurea that usually needs to be taken just once a day, available in 1-, 2-, and 4-milligram sizes.

Repaglinide (Prandin)

Prandin is the first of a new group of drugs called the *meglinitides*. They're chemically unrelated to the sulfonylureas yet work in essentially the same way, which is by stimulating the pancreas to produce more insulin. Experience with repaglinide is limited because it's been available for only a short time, but so far it appears to be quite safe: Its only contraindication is that it should not be used by pregnant or nursing women. Repaglinide comes in 0.5-, 1-, and 2-milligram doses that usually are taken three times daily at least 30 minutes before meals.

Drugs That Have Multiple Effects

But why control glucose levels through just one mode of action if several are possible? That was the thinking behind the development of this multitalented group of drugs known as *biguanides*, only one of which is currently available in the United States.

Metformin (Glucophage)

Metformin was approved by the Food and Drug Administration (FDA) in 1994. The drug has been a real boon in that short time, however, and is often prescribed in addition to other medications (the sulfonylureas, especially) because it has many benefits in addition to its primary one of making cells more insulin sensitive. This dual-purpose medication can help reduce the amount of glucose that enters the bloodstream following meals, and it also can lower the amount of glucose that gets released into the bloodstream by the liver. This is helpful for controlling blood sugar levels not just after meals but between meals and during the night as well.

> *Metformin also can help reduce blood fats as it also acts as an appetite suppressant, thus aiding many type 2 diabetics with the all-important job of losing weight.*

Metformin also can help reduce blood fats (thus lowering the risk of cardiovascular disease) as it also acts as an appetite suppressant, thus aiding many people with type 2 diabetes with the all-important job of losing weight to keep their blood sugar levels under control. Often the drug is prescribed in combination with other type 2 medications, one of the sulfonylureas, especially. It's available in 500-, 850-, and 1,000-milligram tablets and is best taken with meals, two or three times daily. Currently metformin is the most prescribed diabetes drug being used in the United States.

Side effects? As good as metformin is, it is not perfect. It can cause upset stomach, diarrhea, dizziness, weakness, fatigue, a metallic taste in the mouth, and, in rare cases, difficulty breathing. It also has been known to reduce absorption of vitamin B_{12}, an important nutrient for the nervous system and blood. Pregnant or nursing women should not use this drug, nor should heavy drinkers or people with liver disease, kidney disease, or heart failure.

The Thiazolidinediones

The primary action of these drugs, like the biguanides, is to make the body's cells more sensitive to insulin so they can take glucose in for energy. In March 2000, one of the three available thiazolidinediones, troglitizone (Rezulin), was removed from the market by the FDA because it was found to cause serious liver disease in some people, but thus far no such problems have occurred with the two remaining thiazolidinediones discussed here:

- **Rosiglitazone (Avandia)**. A major advantage of this drug is that it needs to be taken only once a day, although it can take as long as 3 months to achieve its maximum effects. Often it is used in conjunction with metformin or one of the sulfonylureas and comes in 2-, 4-, and 8-milligram strengths. The drug can cause water retention leading to swelling of the ankles in some people—older patients, especially—and sometimes is discontinued for this reason. Another drawback is that patients must be tested to be sure they have no signs of liver disease before this drug is prescribed. The drug also has been known to increase fertility in some women of childbearing age.

- **Pioglitizone (Actos)**. This drug is similar to rosiglitazone. It needs to be taken just once daily and can be used along with other type 2 medications, insulin included. It comes in 15-, 30-, and 45-milligram strengths.

Drugs That Reduce Glucose Production

Currently there are two drugs in the category called *alpha-glucosidase inhibitors*—**acarbose (Precose)** and **miglitol (Glyset).** Relatively new, they work by blocking the action of certain key enzymes that help form glucose out of the starches in our diets, thus preventing large amounts of glucose from ever entering the bloodstream at all. This can be especially helpful in preventing glucose surges that can occur after eating. Patients usually are advised to take these medications with the first bite of every meal, although a less frequent schedule initially may be recommended to lessen the chance of unwanted side effects—digestive complaints being the most common. Often these symptoms will begin to subside, however, with continued use.

Precose is available in tablets of 25, 50, or 100 milligrams each. Glyset is available in 25- and 50-milligram strengths.

Two Late Arrivals: Dual-Acting Glucovance and Fast-Acting Starlix

In the fall and then winter of 2000, the FDA approved two more promising new drugs for the treatment of type 2 diabetes: Glucovance and Starlix.

Glyburide with Metformin (Glucovance)

Glucovance is unique in that it combines the pancreas-stimulating effects of a sulfonylurea with metformin, a drug that sensitizes cells to insulin as it also reduces glucose production by the liver. In a study presented at the 60th Scientific Sessions of the American Diabetes Association held in San Antonio, it was reported that type 2 patients receiving Glucovance experienced better glucose control than a group of similar patients given glyburide and metformin separately. The patients also reported fewer gastrointestinal side effects. Because this single drug was more convenient as well as less expensive for patients to use, it could mark the beginning of a new wave of such combination drugs in the future, ADA officials say.

Nateglinide (Starlix)

The other newcomer, Starlix, is the sole member of a new class of type 2 diabetes medications known as *D-phenylalanine derivatives*, which work by rapidly stimulating the pancreas to produce insulin in order to reduce blood sugar increases following meals. It can be used alone or in combination with metformin (Glucophage) and thus far has proven to be highly effective and well tolerated. The most distinguishing characteristic of Starlix is its "fast on, fast off" action, which makes it ideal for meal-related blood sugar control: It works quickly enough to prevent postmeal blood sugar surges but also *stops* working quickly enough to avoid the low blood sugar that can occur with insulin-stimulating drugs that remain active longer. Starlix comes in

Advice on Using Oral Medications

The oral medications for type 2 diabetes, frequently called simply "diabetes pills," are not perfect, nor do they always work well for everyone. But if prescribed in the right combinations and used according to instructions, they can help millions of people with type 2 diabetes live far healthier lives. Generally the pills work best for people who've had diabetes for fewer than 10 years, are not underweight, and who take little or no insulin. Patients should know, too, that these medications may stop working after being effective for months or even years. The reasons are not well understood, but often switching medications or adding a new medication to the mix can help. Women who plan to become pregnant also should know that diabetes pills should not be taken during the gestation period, and many should be avoided during nursing.

Here are some other general recommendations for using these medications with maximum safety as well as effect:

- Diabetes pills should be taken with meals or slightly before them.

- If a dose has been missed, it should not be doubled. Rather, the normal dose should be taken at the next appointed time and the normal schedule resumed.

- Anyone taking diabetes pills should inform his or her doctor of all other medications, prescription as well as over-the-counter, that are being taken.

- Some people taking diabetes pills should be prepared temporarily to switch to insulin injections during times of illness or if a major surgery is required.

60- and 120-milligram strengths and usually is taken with meals three times daily.

HYPOGLYCEMIA: HOW LOW NOT TO GO

Their benefits certainly outweigh their risks, but oral medications for type 2 diabetes that stimulate the pancreas to produce insulin—the sulfonylureas and repaglinide—need to be used exactly as prescribed to prevent a condition known as *hypoglycemia*. Also known simply as "low blood sugar," the condition occurs when glucose levels drop *too low*—below 70 milligrams/deciliter—producing symptoms that can include feeling dizzy or light-headed, nervous and shaky, sleepy or confused, sweaty, or suddenly very hungry. Hypoglycemia can develop when too much medication has been taken for the amount of glucose present in the blood for it to work on.

> *Oral medications for type 2 diabetes that stimulate the pancreas to produce insulin—the sulfonylureas and repaglinide—need to be used exactly as prescribed to prevent hypoglycemia.*

It's important to talk with your doctor right away about your medication schedule if you experience symptoms of hypoglycemia, but you also should be careful to avoid certain situations that can cause the condition. Delaying or skipping a meal, for example, or simply eating too little at a meal can result in low blood sugar. Getting more exercise than usual also can cause the condition, as can drinking alcohol.

The most accurate way to determine whether low blood sugar is causing you to feel suddenly out of sorts is to do a quick glucose monitoring. A reading of below 70 milligrams/deciliter should alert you that yes, your glucose level has dropped too low and that a quick snack containing at least 15 grams of carbohydrate—such as one of the following—should be eaten as soon as possible:

- 1/2 cup of any fruit juice
- 1/2 cup of regular (not diet) soda

- 1 cup of milk or skim milk
- 1 or 2 teaspoons of sugar or honey
- 5 or 6 pieces of hard candy
- Glucose gel or tablets equaling 15 grams of carbohydrate

Test your glucose levels 15 minutes after you've eaten one of these foods or a carbohydrate equivalent, and if your blood sugar still is below 70 milligrams/deciliter, have another 15 grams of carbohydrate and test yourself again. If your glucose still is too low and you're still not feeling well, call your doctor. Severe cases of hypoglycemia can lead to coma and even death.

INSULIN: THE FIRST AND STILL FOREMOST

Insulin was the first diabetes medication, developed by two Canadian doctors in the early 1920s, and for people with type 1 diabetes, it remains the only one. "Without daily insulin injections, most people with type 1 diabetes would die within 72 to 96 hours," Dr. Bernstein says. This is because insulin is the vital link between the food we eat and nourishment we derive from it. When insulin is not available in adequate amounts, food (in the form of glucose) "sits on the table," in a sense, but the body's cells don't have the required "silverware" (insulin) to consume it.

Yes, It's for Type 2, Too

But isn't insulin needed only by people with type 1 diabetes?

"Certainly not," Dr. Bernstein says. "Somewhere between 30 and 40 percent of people with type 2 diabetes require insulin therapy, and especially as they get older, or if their conditions are not being well managed in other ways, such as with diet and exercise or oral medications."

Consider Barbara, for example, who, at a recent meeting with her doctor, reacted with a mixture of anger and surprise when told her

Aspirin and Diabetes: A Match for the Heart's Content

Known already to reduce heart attacks in the general population, aspirin now is being recognized for being especially beneficial for diabetics. Taking just a single baby aspirin a day can reduce risks for heart attacks in people with diabetes by as much as 60 percent, according to the *American Diabetes Association Complete Guide to Diabetes.* Aspirin exerts its protective effect mostly by reducing the "stickiness" of blood platelets that have been exposed to excess glucose, thus decreasing their tendency to adhere to blood vessel walls—a process that can lay the foundation not just for heart attacks but also strokes, the ADA says.

The ADA recommends that unless contraindicated for other medical reasons, aspirin should be taken daily by people with either type 1 or type 2 diabetes who have known heart disease and also by those without heart disease if they smoke, are overweight, have high blood pressure or high cholesterol, or have a parent or sibling who has suffered a heart attack before the age of 50. For most people, as little as a single baby aspirin a day is enough to exert aspirin's protective effects, research shows, but some people who are less re-

treatment for type 2 diabetes would have to be changed. "But wait a minute," she said. "Didn't you tell me less than a year ago when we discovered my blood sugar problems that insulin probably wouldn't be necessary?"

Her doctor agreed that had been true, but he also informed Barbara that she had gained 10 pounds instead of losing the 10 he had recommended and that she hadn't been very diligent about taking her medications as he had prescribed them, either. So now insulin was necessary, a choice that had been hers to make.

Such scenes play out all-too often, Dr. Bernstein says, and what they point to is a major stumbling block in type 2 treatment. "Many

sponsive to aspirin may need to take an adult-sized tablet of 325 milligrams, the ADA notes.

To reduce risks of stomach irritation, especially in people over 60, the ADA recommends taking aspirin with an *enteric* coating, which causes the medication to break down in the intestines rather than in the stomach. Taking aspirin with food is another way to reduce its risks of causing stomach irritation, the ADA says.

Also be sure to check with your doctor before taking aspirin if you have any doubts it might not be safe for you. It could be dangerous if you have a stomach ulcer, for example, or liver disease. There are other medications—the prescription drugs ticlopidine and clopidogrel, for example—that can duplicate aspirin's beneficial effects. Also check with your doctor to make sure you're not taking any other medications that could react with aspirin adversely.

Note: Don't assume that all over-the-counter painkillers contain aspirin, because unless a product specifies aspirin on its label, chances are it does not. Such common pain remedies as acetaminophen (Tylenol), ibuprofen (Motrin, Advil), and naproxen sodium (Aleve) contain pain-reducing ingredients other than aspirin and will not have aspirin's same heart-healthy effects.

patients simply don't give type 2 diabetes the respect it deserves in terms of how serious it can be," he says. "It's not uncommon for type 2 patients to disregard treatment recommendations entirely, in fact. Rather than give up the foods they love or lose weight or start working out, they say they'd rather just take their chances."

And chances are those chances are not very good. "In my 30 years of treating type 2 diabetes, I've never seen a remission or even anything close," Dr. Bernstein says. "It's a whole different story, of course, if people begin to change the way they live and correct things that may be contributing to their disease, but otherwise type 2 diabetes will always just get worse."

New and Improved

With a prognosis like this, it certainly makes sense to listen up if it seems insulin may be needed. Yes, it needs to be injected, but new innovations can now make the process nearly painless. And yes, the injections may need to be done several times a day, but that can become a matter of habit. And yes, insulin can be expensive, but new programs now are making that less painful, too.

> *Many patients simply don't give type 2 diabetes the respect it deserves in terms of how serious it can be.*
>
> —GERALD BERNSTEIN, M.D.

The most important thing is that insulin can work. Not many discoveries in the field of medicine are praised as lifesaving "breakthroughs," but insulin has been one of them. "One of the greatest medical achievements of all time," says Richard S. Beaser, M.D., an assistant clinical professor of medicine at Harvard Medical School and chair of the Patient Education Committee at the esteemed Joslin Diabetes Center in Boston.

Insulin, remember, is the key needed to unlock the doors that allow the entry of glucose into the body's cells. It's a naturally occurring substance made by the pancreas, but up until 1978, the only way scientists could produce insulin for medicinal use was by extracting it from the pancreas of animals, usually cows and pigs. Because these preparations were difficult to purify completely, some patients experienced adverse reactions to them, which could vary from slight redness and itching at the site of injection to considerable swelling and pain. The immune systems of some patients, moreover, worked to reject animal insulin entirely, producing antibodies to defend against what their bodies perceived to be an invasion of foreign pathogens, thus rendering the insulin less effective.

Modern techniques eliminated many of these problems with animal insulin, and it remained in use by many patients for decades. Today, however, all insulins produced in the United States are human insulin or synthetic insulins, chemically similar to human insulin but produced by genetic engineering, and totally free of the adverse reac-

Easing the Financial Strain

Diabetes medications can be expensive, and possibly your insurance plan doesn't provide adequate coverage. If that's true, you may be eligible to receive medications free of charge from several pharmaceutical companies that offer patient assistance programs. To qualify, you'll need a prescription from your doctor showing the medications you require, and your doctor also will need to fill out a special form indicating that you are, in fact, in financial need.

Here are some companies currently offering such programs along with the drugs they offer and the phone numbers to call for information on how to apply.

Company	Medication	Program	Phone
Bayer Corporation	acarbose	Indigent Patient	(800) 998-9180
Bristol Meyers	metformin	Patient Assistance	(800) 437-0994
Eli Lilly and Company	insulin	Lilly Cares	(800) 545-6962
Aventis	glyburide, glimepiride	Indigent Patient	(800) 221-4025
Novo Nordisk	insulin	Indigent Program	(800) 727-6500
Parke Davis	troglitizone	Patient Assistance	(908) 725-1247
Pfizer	glipizide, chlorpropamide	Pfizer Prescription Assistance	(800) 646-4455

tions formerly associated with the older types. Another major advance in insulin therapy has been the development of several types of medications that take action at different speeds and remain active for different lengths of time—some, like the recently developed glargine insulin, for as long as 24 hours. This allows patients far greater flexibility in controlling blood sugar levels in ways that correspond more closely to their particular lifestyles. Unlike before, when there was just one type of insulin that worked at one speed and usually had to be injected several times a day, insulin now is available in short-, intermediate-, and long-acting varieties that differ in these three important ways:

> *A*nother major advance in insulin therapy has been the development of several types of medications that take action at different speeds and remain active for different lengths of time.

1. **Onset.** The amount of time required for the insulin to become active in lowering glucose levels.

2. **Peak time.** The length of time the insulin works at peak efficiency.

3. **Duration.** The length of time the insulin is active, even if not at peak efficiency.

WORTH A SHOT

Insulin therapy for type 2 diabetes may be needed at any stage if other methods to control blood sugar fail to do an adequate job, but not until later stages of the disease is it usually required. This may be caused by a continued deterioration of the insulin-producing beta cells of the pancreas, further development of insulin resistance on the part of the body's cells, or an increase in glucose contribution by the liver. Whatever the reason, if your doctor decides insulin is the answer, it's a decision you'll need to respect because delivering insulin therapy, remember, is a task that must be performed by *you*. Is it worth it?

"Absolutely," Dr. Bernstein says. "Insulin therapy remains the most direct and effective method for controlling blood sugar levels in type 1 and type 2 patients alike, and it could save thousands of lives every year if it were only more widely used." Until recently, injection by syringe was the only delivery method available, but there are now devices that make the process easier as well as less painful. But more on those in a minute. Let's look first at the different types of insulin now available:

- **Long-acting ultralente insulin.** The advantage of this insulin is that, although it can take as long as 6 hours to begin working, it provides a low-level yet still active supply of insulin for as long as 26 hours, permitting some people to get by with just one injection a day. In the spring of 2000, moreover, the FDA approved another long-acting insulin called *insulin glargine* (Lantus), which stays active for a full 24 hours yet goes to work quickly (usually within just 2 hours) and exerts its glucose control in a steady, "peak-free" manner similar to the way the pancreas releases insulin naturally. The new insulin is expected to be a highly effective addition to the long-acting insulin arsenal.

- **Intermediate-acting NPH or lente insulin.** These insulins usually begin working within 1 to 3 hours of injection and generally will continue to be active for 16 to 24 hours, thus assuring that at least some insulin is active in the body at all times during a 24-hour period.

- **Short-acting regular insulin.** This is the type of insulin that was used for decades before the others were developed. It becomes active within about 30 minutes, reaches peak activity at about 3 hours, and usually will have finished working after about 8 hours.

- **Rapid-acting lispro insulin.** This is the latest addition to the insulin lineup, and it's been a very valuable one because its quick action can be helpful in controlling glucose levels in response to meals. Lispro insulin is active within just 5 minutes, reaches peak efficiency after about 1 hour, and ceases activity after 3 hours. This means the insulin can be taken at the first bite of a meal and still be active in time for the digestive process.

- **Premixed insulins**. These medications usually will be a combination of a regular, short-acting insulin and a longer-acting, intermediate one so that a wide range of glucose control can be achieved with just a single insulin injection.

Insulin Essentials

Whatever type of insulin you may be prescribed, here are some pointers for using and storing the medication that are common to all:

- **Injection site**. How quickly insulin begins working will be affected by where it's injected: It works fastest when injected in the area of the abdomen, more slowly when injected into the arms, and slowest of all when injected into the buttocks or thighs. The depth of injection also will affect how quickly insulin becomes active: The deeper the injection, the faster the action. Know, too, that insulin injections will take effect sooner—and have a greater effect—when followed by exercise.

- **Allergic reaction**. Because of ingredients added to retard spoilage or prolong their activity, even the new and much-improved human insulins can cause allergic reactions in some people. Usually such disturbances will occur at the time and site of injection and may take the form of swelling, redness, dents under the skin, or small bumps similar to hives. If you experience any of these reactions, check right away with your doctor.

- **Storage**. Insulin may be stored at room temperature for as long as 4 weeks or in a refrigerator until the expiration date on the label. Do not allow insulin to be exposed to sunlight or extreme heat or cold.

- **To be thrifty**. Disposable syringes are designed to be used just once and then discarded, but to save money, it's generally okay to "break the rules" and get two or three uses out of a syringe before throwing it out. If you decide to do this, be sure to recap the syringe and keep it in a clean, dry place out of the reach of children. Also try to use the syringe within 24 hours.

- **Disposal**. When it does come time to dispose of a syringe, do so responsibly. Collect your used syringes in a puncture-proof container with a lid, and dispose of them according to the regulations for medical waste in your area.

- **In a pinch**. It's not recommended, but insulin injections may be given safely through clothing.

INJECTING INSULIN: THE BASIC DRILL

If the idea of injecting insulin seems to you a fate as unfortunate as diabetes itself, take comfort in knowing that the procedure at least is a lot less inconvenient or painful than it used to be. Not only are there new devices that simplify the process immensely, even the equipment used for injecting insulin the old-fashioned way has been greatly improved. Needles are now thinner with sharper points and special lubricated coatings that enter the skin more smoothly. If you're using the latest equipment and your injections still cause you a lot of pain, check with your doctor or diabetes educator. You may need to make some changes in your injection technique, or you may simply need to relax: Tense muscles can increase the hurt.

Recommended sites for injection include the abdomen (where insulin is absorbed the fastest), the upper buttocks, the backs of the arms, and front of the thighs (see figure 3.1). To avoid unnecessary irritation or pain, these sites should be rotated so that the same site is never injected consecutively. Repeated injections in one area can cause a buildup of fat and fibrous tissue called *hypertrophy* that can limit insulin absorption in addition to causing greater discomfort.

How often you need to inject and the type of insulin you use will depend on your particular condition and lifestyle, and these details

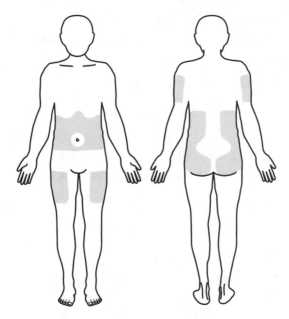

Figure 3.1—*Injection Sites*

will be specified by your doctor. You also will be given instructions on how to deliver your injections, but we'll give you the basics of the procedure again here in the event you should need a quick review:

1. If the insulin you plan to use has been in the refrigerator, warm the bottle by rolling it between the palms of your hands for a minute or so: Injecting insulin that's cold can cause more pain.

2. Clean the site you intend to inject with soap and water or a quick swipe of rubbing alcohol. (Be sure to let the rubbing alcohol dry, however, because your injection will cause a greater stinging sensation if you don't.)

3. With the syringe in your right hand (if you're right-handed), use your left hand to pinch an inch or so of skin between your forefinger and thumb.

4. With a quick thrust, and holding the syringe as you would a dart, insert the needle at an angle of between 45 and 90 degrees.

Speed is of the essence here, because, like removing an adhesive bandage, the faster your motion, the less pain you'll feel. And don't be afraid to insert the needle as deep as it will go, which with most of the new shorter needles will be only about $5/16$ inch.

5. Once penetration has been made, press the plunger on the syringe to deliver the insulin dose, then pull the syringe out.

Note: The angle at which you make your injection should depend on the amount of fat you're injecting into. For most people with type 2 diabetes, ample fat is not a problem, so an insertion angle of 90 degrees—which will represent a straight-on, perpendicular thrust—is best. If you are thin, however, making your injection at a 45-degree angle may be preferable to keep the needle from penetrating muscle tissue or even bone (see figure 3.2).

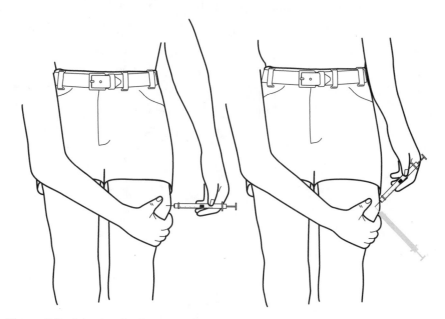

Figure 3.2—*Injection Angles: 90 and 45 Degrees*

INJECTION ALTERNATIVES: LIFESAVERS FOR THE SQUEAMISH

Scientists have been concerned not just about the health of people with diabetes, thankfully, but also their comfort. They've come up with alternatives to the standard needle and syringe for injecting insulin, and the devices are making life a lot easier for millions of type 1 and type 2 patients. If any of the following approaches sound interesting, check to see whether your doctor has a sample of the device you could inspect before deciding to buy one. Also ask whether your doctor thinks the device would be appropriate for your particular condition and lifestyle.

- **Insulin pumps.** These devices provide a steady flow of insulin to the body by way of a tube inserted in the skin, usually in the area of the abdomen. The pump portion, weighing a mere 4 ounces and no bigger than a paging device, is worn on the belt (see figure 3.3). Although expensive at $3,000 to $5,000, the

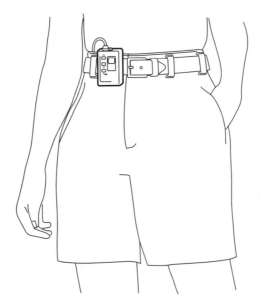

Figure 3.3—*Insulin Pump*

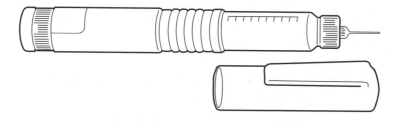

Figure 3.4—*Insulin Pen*

units do a very good job of providing a smooth insulin supply and even allow for sudden increases of insulin to be delivered for occasions such as the increased insulin demands of meals. The pumps, which can hold a 1- or 2-day supply of insulin without having to be refilled, are most suited for type 1 patients who must inject insulin regularly and often.

- **Pen injectors.** As their name implies, these devices resemble a fountain pen, with a disposable needle serving as its "writing tip" and a small cartridge containing insulin instead of ink (see figure 3.4). You simply set the size of the dose of insulin to be delivered using a small dial that makes a clicking sound (especially useful in helping the visually impaired set their dosage amount) and then simply give yourself a quick poke. The pens are convenient to use and also highly accurate in delivering insulin in specified amounts. Most people in Europe who use insulin now use this method of delivery.

- **Jet injectors.** These ingenious devices manage to get insulin into the bloodstream without any needle at all. With just the press of a button, insulin is forced into the skin by a powerful blast of air emitted from the tip of the device, usually with little if any discomfort for the patient (see figure 3.5). The units can cost in the neighborhood of $1,000, but for people morbidly afraid of needles—or for administering insulin to small children—they can very quickly earn their keep.

Getting Insurance to Pay

Because every insurance plan is different, it's impossible to say what portion, if any, of the cost of diabetes supplies will be covered by your particular program. If you encounter resistance to being reimbursed for a device such as an insulin injector or insulin pump, however, do not necessarily accept no for an answer. "Keep asking," advise the editors of *American Diabetes Association Complete Guide to Diabetes.* Your best requests are made in well-written letters, explaining the results of the Diabetes Control and Complications Trial, which found that tight glucose control definitely works to reduce long-term complications of this disease, and how such reductions stand to benefit everyone—your insurance company included.

Ask your doctor and diabetes educator to support you by writing letters of their own, making the same point and explaining the benefits of tight glucose control in your particular case.

At one time, most insurance companies would not pay for therapeutic footwear for people with diabetes, the editors of *American Diabetes Association Complete Guide to Diabetes* point out, but pressure from doctors and their patients induced them to change their stance. Similar progress, with the right push from patients and their doctors, stands to be made regarding other coverage issues.

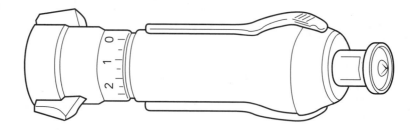

Figure 3.5—*Jet Injector*

- **Spring-loaded injector aids.** These devices allow patients to deliver their injections simply by pushing a button. The button activates a spring-loaded device that forces the needle into the skin in just a fraction of a second. This makes the injection process not only less painful, but also much easier for people such as arthritis patients who may have limited use of their hands.

- **Infusers.** With this innovation, insulin is injected not directly into the skin but rather into a small tube that has been inserted beneath the skin, usually in the area of the abdomen. The tube needs to be removed and relocated every 2 or 3 days, unfortunately, but many patients consider the system preferable to regular insulin injections.

For more information on insulin delivery products, including local suppliers and costs, contact your local ADA branch, or check in the back of the ADA's magazine *Diabetes Forecast*. The ADA also publishes a catalog, *The Buyer's Guide to Diabetes Supplies*. Contact your local chapter or call (800) 232-6733 to obtain a copy.

CHAPTER 4

Glucose Monitoring
The Key to Glucose Mastery

❧

Monitoring. The word itself sounds passive and unimportant—more like watching something rather than acting on it. But when it comes to the erratic glucose levels and other potential complications of diabetes, *monitoring* is the key to *mastery*. Only by watching the ups and downs of blood sugar levels can you learn their patterns and gather the information needed to control them. "Trying to treat diabetes without regular monitoring of glucose levels," says former American Diabetes Association (ADA) president Gerald Bernstein, M.D., "is like trying to cross the street with your eyes closed."

Yet millions of people with diabetes, unfortunately, are trying to do just that. According to a recent study, 20 percent of people with diabetes do no self-testing of their blood sugar levels at all. And when it comes to following all five of the monitoring goals currently recommended for proper diabetes care (described later), the number of faithful adherents slips to less than 3 percent.

We'll be looking at the doctor-assisted tests later in this chapter. But mainly we'll be looking at the testing that only you can do, the self-monitoring for blood glucose (SMBG, as it's called) that can tell

Doing Lousy, Feeling Fine

With a lot of illnesses, what you see is what you get. Catch a cold or flu, for example, and you're going to be sneezing, wheezing, aching, and feeling bad pretty much from head to toe. Not so with diabetes. This disease can be doing considerable damage while leaving us feeling fine. Many people with diabetes find this surprising because they think they can sense when their blood sugar levels are high or low, but with the exception of extreme levels, usually they cannot.

This is why regular glucose monitoring is so important, and to prevent not just the long-term complications of glucose levels being too high but also the short-term dangers of blood sugar levels falling too low, a common problem for people being treated with insulin or oral medications that cause the pancreas to increase its insulin output. Called *hypoglycemia,* low blood sugar can be especially perilous because it can cause lapses in the very mental capabilities required for someone to know that it has occurred. People can become so disoriented so quickly when stricken with low blood sugar that they quite literally don't know what has hit them—very dangerous indeed during activities such as driving, operating power equipment, or even just caring for young children. Hypoglycemia can cause extreme mental confusion, muscular weakness, dizziness, rapid heartbeat, irritability, and a tingling sensation in the face or lips. If untreated, it can cause loss of consciousness and even death.

On the flip side are the dangers of high blood sugar levels, known as *hyperglycemia,* which also can come on in a flash. Hyperglycemia can be triggered by missing an insulin injection or dose of oral med-

you how your blood sugar levels are behaving—or misbehaving—on a day-to-day and even hourly basis. The information provided by frequent self-monitoring is invaluable in helping both you and your health care team maximize the effects of your treatment program, but too often this testing simply doesn't get done. Some patients fail to

ication but also by such natural occurrences as illness, stress, or simply eating too much. If in excess of approximately 250 milligrams/deciliter, elevated blood sugar levels usually will be noticeable—producing symptoms such as stomach pains, vomiting, blurred vision, feelings of weakness, intense thirst, facial flushing, or difficulty breathing—but such extreme levels are relatively rare. Far more common, and insidious, are moderately elevated levels in the 140 to 240 milligrams/deciliter range because these usually will not produce noticeable signs, allowing us to feel well when we are not. Levels in this range are high enough to be doing internal damage, but not high enough to cause us to take action, and therein lies their danger.

Glucose monitoring to the rescue. By letting you know the truth about your blood sugar levels—whether you feel well or not—regular glucose monitoring can give you and your health care team the information you need to keep your blood sugar levels as stable as possible. Without such monitoring, your diabetes could be tricking you into thinking all is well when things most definitely are not. "That's the danger with this disease," Dr. Gerald Bernstein says. "It does some of its greatest damage through deception, letting us feel fine as it slowly whittles away at some of our most vital tissues."

Diabetes, in short, is one case where what you don't know definitely *can* hurt you. Don't risk it. Test your blood sugar levels at least twice daily if you have type 2 diabetes and at least four times daily (before meals and once before bed) if you have type 1 or are a type 2 patient taking insulin. Like the watched pot that won't boil, diabetes won't brew up its cauldron of woe if you keep it under such a watchful eye.

understand the importance; others simply won't endure the inconvenience. Either way, diabetes needlessly continues on its rampage. Read on, and learn how monitoring your glucose levels regularly can be the single most important effort you make—in just a few minutes a day—to help stop this rampage even before it starts.

WHY TREATMENT IS NOT ENOUGH

Paula could accept being diagnosed with type 2 diabetes, and at 5 feet, 3 inches and 180 pounds, she was willing to assume some of the responsibility. She was even okay with the treatment plan of weight loss, exercise, and oral medication spelled out for her by her doctor. It was the self-testing for glucose levels she was told she'd have to do—daily!—she was having a problem with.

> *The information provided by frequent self-monitoring is invaluable in helping both you and your health care team maximize the effects of your treatment program.*

"If I'm doing everything I'm supposed to be doing, why should I need to test myself?" she asked her doctor. "Is it because all the things you're telling me to do might not work? That's certainly not very encouraging."

Paula's quandary is a common one and a considerable stumbling block to the successful treatment of type 1 and 2 diabetes alike. Maybe you've even wondered about the value of glucose monitoring yourself. If treatment works, after all, why should it be so important to be on the lookout for evidence that it's *not* working?

To answer that, it can help to take a journey inside the body to see why glucose levels in someone with diabetes take such a wild, up-and-down ride in the first place. In the normal body, blood sugar levels remain relatively constant 24 hours a day, rarely deviating by more than about 70 points or exceeding approximately 140 milligrams/deciliter. In someone with diabetes, however, glucose levels can surge to heights approaching 1,000 milligrams/deciliter, and within just a few minutes. (See table 1 for desirable glucose levels.) That's the kind of volatility treatment has to control, and it's not an easy job. In the normal body, glucose control is accomplished automatically and naturally as rising glucose levels in the blood cue the release of just the right amount of insulin from the pancreas. The body's cells use the insulin to allow the glucose entry, and all goes smoothly. Not so in the diabetic body, however.

Table 1. Desirable Glucose Levels

	Fasting and Before Meals	2 Hours After Meals
People without diabetes	80–120 mg/dl	100–140 mg/dl
Ideal ranges for people with diabetes	80–120 mg/dl	100–140 mg/dl
Acceptable ranges for people with diabetes	80–120 mg/dl	Up to 160 mg/dl
Acceptable ranges for pregnant women with diabetes	65–95 mg/dl	Less than 120 mg/dl

What the normal body does naturally to control glucose levels, the diabetic body needs help to do, and that's why regular self-testing for glucose is so critical. Self-testing takes on the role of the pancreas, essentially, assessing the amount of glucose in the blood so that the right amount of insulin can be injected, or the right doses of oral medications can be taken, to keep glucose levels from taking their wild rides. Self-testing also is important for providing the information needed for dietary and exercise programs to be used as effectively as possible for glucose control. As Dr. Bernstein points out, without regular testing for glucose levels, all of our potentially most effective strategies for treating diabetes—insulin, oral medications, diet, and exercise—become little better than shots in the dark.

For these reasons, all people with diabetes should set the following five monitoring goals:

1. Self-testing for glucose levels several times daily (before meals and bedtime)

2. At least four doctor visits a year if on insulin and two if not

3. At least four hemoglobin A1c tests done annually

4. At least four examinations of the feet each year

5. At least one examination of the eyes each year

CONTROL TODAY, HEALTH TOMORROW

As we learned in chapter 1, diabetes is not a disease we can afford to treat in a hit-or-miss fashion. Every time blood sugar levels sneak out of control, they take a little piece of our health along with them, and we can't get that health back. Unlike a clogged artery that can be re-paired or a cancerous tumor that can be surgi-cally removed, giving us a "clean slate," the effects of even a single surge of high blood sugar can tarnish our health in ways that we must live with for the rest of our lives. Hence the unques-tionable wisdom in doing everything possible—including regular glucose monitoring—not to let these surges occur in the first place.

> *What the normal body does natu-rally to control glucose levels, the diabetic body needs help to do, and that's where regular self-testing for glucose becomes so critical.*

Remember that in the Diabetes Control and Complications Trial (DCCT) mentioned in chapter 1, it was the people who monitored their blood sugars most closely who earned the best results—reducing their risks of some complications by as much as 76 percent. What the DCCT showed is that the high blood sugar you avoid today can help lay the foundation for the better health you can expect tomorrow, and long after that. What your future will look like with this disease de-pends on what you do today, in the present. With the help of regular glucose monitoring, that future can be very bright, indeed.

"In so many ways, what you reap is what you sow with diabetes," Dr. Bernstein reminds us. "The disease can control the patient or the patient can control the disease, and glucose monitoring is at the very core of where that control begins. Monitoring provides the information on which treatment needs to be based. Only by finding out where treatment may be failing, after all, can we learn how to make it succeed."

Please consider the following guidelines for self-testing for blood glucose with that crucial point in mind. Only by knowing why and when glucose levels "misbehave" can we organize and execute and the most effective strategies for keeping them in line. Yes, scientists have given us many highly effective medications for helping regulate blood sugar levels, as we saw in chapter 3, and it's also true that diet and exercise and a growing number of alternative therapies also can do a great job of helping keep glucose levels

> *The ever-changing glucose levels characteristic of diabetes should be thought of us as a moving target: The more we can learn their patterns, the more accurately our treatments can be aimed.*

under control, as we'll be seeing in chapters 5 and 6. But without regular testing of the effects of these strategies, they're going to miss the all-important mark. The ever-changing glucose levels characteristic of diabetes should be thought of us as a moving target: The more we can learn their patterns, the more accurately our treatments can be aimed.

WHO NEEDS TO TEST, AND WHEN

The editors of *The American Diabetes Association Complete Guide to Diabetes* make it very clear: The key to achieving long-term goals in glucose control is to pursue short-term goals. If you can manage your glucose levels just one day at a time, the bigger picture will take care of itself. Here are the ADA's current recommendations for who should self-test for glucose levels and how often:

> **People with type 1 diabetes and people with type 2 taking insulin.** Glucose should be tested before each meal and at bedtime every day, with an additional fifth test during the middle of the

night (at about 3 A.M.) once a week. If that sounds like a lot, rest assured that studies have shown a relationship between the number of tests done a day and the level of glucose control. When the number of tests decreases to below four a day, glucose control decreases as well.

People with type 2 diabetes taking oral medications. Glucose should be tested at least twice a day—once before breakfast and again before dinner—and preferably three times, with an additional test before bedtime. More frequent testing may be advised early in a treatment program, however, as an additional aid in establishing the best medication schedule.

People with type 2 diabetes who control their diabetes with just diet and exercise. As with type 2 patients taking medications, glucose should be tested twice a day, before breakfast and again before dinner, until a program of diet and exercise is found that keeps glucose levels stable. After that period, testing may be reduced to three or four times a week as long as the treatment program continues to be effective.

Women with gestational diabetes. Diabetes during pregnancy requires the most frequent glucose monitoring of all because high glucose levels can do irreparable harm to the fetus. Talk to your doctor about the schedule that would be best for you given your particular condition.

WHAT THE TESTS SHOW

If glucose monitoring is so critical, what sort of information can these tests actually reveal, and how can this information be used to help you structure your treatment program? That depends on whether insulin injections are part of your therapy. Let's first look at the benefits of testing for people using insulin, then the benefits for people who do not.

For People Using Insulin

A common injection schedule for type 1 patients, and also type 2 patients requiring insulin, is to inject a mixture of a fast-acting and intermediate-acting insulin twice a day—one dosage before breakfast and another before dinner. Here's what testing for someone on that schedule can show:

The before-breakfast test. This test shows whether the amount of intermediate-acting insulin injected the previous day before dinner has been sufficient to maintain satisfactory blood sugar levels throughout the night.

The before-lunch test. This test indicates whether the short-acting insulin injected before breakfast has been adequate for the period between breakfast and lunch.

The before-dinner test. This test reveals whether the intermediate-acting insulin administered before breakfast has been enough for the hours between lunch and dinner.

The before-bedtime test. This test shows whether the short-acting insulin injected before the evening meal has been adequate for the period between dinner and bedtime.

For People Not Using Insulin

If you have type 2 diabetes and are not taking oral medication, you may be asked to monitor your glucose levels once or twice a day. Here's why:

The before-breakfast test. This test will show whether the amount of insulin produced by your body has been sufficient to maintain satisfactory glucose levels throughout the previous night.

The after-dinner test. This test will show whether the insulin your body has been producing has been enough to control the blood sugar levels that normally rise after your evening meal.

Note: Because medication schedules and treatment programs vary widely for each patient, these testing regimens may not be appropriate for you. These schedules are offered here only as examples of the kind of useful information glucose monitoring can provide. Be sure to check with your doctor or leader of your health care team to determine the schedule that is most suited for your particular needs.

THE VALUE OF ADDITIONAL TESTS: MORE "LETTERS ON THE BOARD"

In addition to testing your glucose levels at the times recommended by your doctor, it can be useful to test at other times to get as complete a picture as possible of your overall blood sugar "personality." Consider monitoring your glucose levels as being a bit like playing the TV game show *Wheel of Fortune*. The more you test, the more "letters" you put on the board, and hence the more information you and your health care team will have to go on in putting together the best treatment possible for solving your particular diabetes puzzle.

That can be a helpful notion to keep in mind if you're feeling short on the kind of motivation that frequent monitoring may require. You're not just amassing meaningless numbers, you should remind yourself, you're putting more "letters" on your board, bringing a "solution" to your blood sugar problem that much closer with every drop of blood you draw. Do your best to test at these other times with that in mind:

- **Test when you're ill**. Most illnesses cause glucose levels to go up, but you can't know by how much or for how long unless you test.

- **Test before and after exercise**. Exercise generally causes glucose to go down, but as with an illness, you can't know how far or for how long unless you test.

- **Test when you've eaten something unusual**. Curious about the effects of your mother-in-law's much-acclaimed shepherd's pie? You won't know unless you test.

- **Test when you try a new medication**. Whether it's a prescription drug or simply an over-the-counter cold medication or painkiller, it could have an effect on your blood sugar, but only by testing can you know for sure.

- **Test when you're angry or stressed**. Had a bad day at the office or bout of road rage on the way home? A test is apt to reveal a rise in glucose along with your temper.

- **Test when you're tipsy**. What effect does alcohol have on blood sugar? Again, test and find out. Usually alcohol will drive blood sugar down, especially on an empty stomach. But a sugar-laden aperitif following a piece of Boston cream pie may have a different effect entirely. Only by testing can you know for sure.

- **Test before you drive**. This can be especially important if you suspect low blood sugar may be a problem, the effects of which can come on suddenly and make driving very hazardous. If you do get readings that are low, be sure to correct them before as much as looking for your keys.

Don't Just Test—Record

This goes for all the glucose monitoring you do. The reason for these tests, remember, is to help you recognize patterns to your extreme ups and downs, so that you can learn the best ways to prevent them. You should be able to get a special type of "score sheet" for keeping detailed records of the results of your tests from your doctor, or often such data sheets will be included with whatever type of glucose meter you decide to use. Whatever recording system you use, be sure it includes at least as much information as the sample monitoring chart shown in figure 4.1.

Why Frequent Testing Is Best

Again, in the interest of providing your health care team with the most accurate information, it's wise to consider that several factors

Date	Glucose Test Results					Insulin						
	Before Breakfast	Before Noon Meal	Before Supper	At Bedtime	Other	Regular	Long/ Intermediate	Regular	Regular	Long/ Intermediate	Regular	Long/ Intermediate

Figure 4.1—*Diabetes Monitoring Chart*

contribute to your unique condition, as the preceding list suggests. If you're taking insulin or an oral medication—or some combination of the two—both the amount and timing of your dosages have to be coordinated with several lifestyle variables. Let's take a closer look at some of the variables in the mix.

The Type and Amount of Food You Eat

Glucose levels rise in response to meals, usually peaking about 1 to 2 hours after a meal is over, but how much glucose levels rise will depend both on the amount and type of food eaten. Starchy and sugary foods high in carbohydrates will have a greater and faster effect on glucose levels than foods high in protein or fat. To properly match the timing and amount of insulin or medication you use, therefore, you need to know as specifically as possible what these effects will be— and glucose monitoring is the way. It may be necessary, especially in the beginning of a treatment program when the best medication schedule needs to be determined, to test before and then again about an hour after eating to get as good an idea as possible of what you can expect your glucose responses to be.

The Intensity and Duration of the Exercise You Do

While food drives glucose up, physical activity tends to pull it down, because working muscles use glucose for fuel. But as with meals, the magnitude of this effect will depend on the exercise. The longer the activity, the more glucose it will tend to require, and hence the lower your glucose levels will go when the exercise is complete. Short, strenuous bouts of exercise such as weight-lifting, vigorous swimming, or fast running can actually raise glucose levels, however, by activating glycogen, a form of glucose stored in the muscles and liver. The variable effects of exercise can be further compounded depending on what's been eaten and when—yet more reason to test yourself after a workout to see where your glucose levels stand. To get the true effects of an exercise session, however, wait 1 to 2 hours after you've finished (providing you haven't eaten anything during that time) because it can take that long for glucose levels to stabilize. Much of the glucose muscles use for fuel comes from what they keep stored, and it can take 2 hours or so for them to draw the glucose they need from the blood to replenish their reserves.

The Amount of Stress You Endure, and How You Endure It

Stress, whether emotional or physical, can add yet another variable to the already delicate blood sugar equation. While stressful events can raise glucose levels in some people, they can lower glucose levels in others, so it's a good idea to test yourself to see where you stand in this regard. The blood sugar fluctuations caused by stress are thought to be due to how the body reacts to the release of the hormone epinephrine (also called *adrenaline*), which mobilizes glucose stored in the muscles and liver. The reason for the extra glucose is to prepare the body for the "fight or flight" response, an evolutionary holdover from our less civilized days when life was often punctuated by needs either to defend ourselves from an adversary or to flee from it. Today, unfortunately, we can rarely resolve our conflicts so decisively, which can lead to symptoms such as chronic headaches, anxiety disorders, high blood pressure, and even elevated blood fats. None of these is healthy for anyone, much less someone suffering from diabetes, so if you think stress may be a problem for you, talk to your health care team about getting some help. The stress of dealing with your disease is enough without life itself adding to your load.

> *To get the true effects of an exercise session, wait 1 to 2 hours after you've finished because it can take that long for glucose levels to stabilize.*

Illness or Infection

An illness—even something as minor as a cold or sore throat—can raise glucose levels in addition to increasing insulin resistance on the part of the body's cells, a double-whammy that makes it doubly important to check your blood sugar levels often when an illness or an infection strikes. Illnesses and infections boost blood sugar levels for the same reason as does emotional stress: The body releases hormones that activate glucose stored in the liver as fuel for dealing with the crisis. These same hormones also tend to block the action of insulin, so glucose levels in the blood can rise in a hurry. Glucose can become even more concentrated in the blood due to dehydration if the illness is one that causes fluid loss through diarrhea or vomiting, so you should be especially diligent to monitor your levels if these unpleasantries occur.

> *Illnesses and infections boost blood sugar levels for the same reason as emotional stress: The body releases hormones that activate glucose stored in the liver.*

The Dawn Phenomenon

Yet another anomaly to be aware of is the tendency for blood sugar levels to be high in the morning when you awake. Doctors refer to it as the "dawn phenomenon," seeing it as a natural consequence of the body's circadian rhythms that cause blood sugar levels to rise as a kind of wake-up call for the new day. Don't be alarmed by these high readings, but do check with your doctor on how they should best be handled.

Inconsistency Within Yourself

As if all these intangibles weren't enough, how your body reacts to them day-to-day can vary as well, which increases the importance of frequent testing even more. The more often you test, the better your understanding of your condition, and hence the more effective your treatment is going to be.

HOW TO TEST: DON'T LET PRACTICE MAKE IMPERFECT

So monitoring glucose levels is the key to mastering glucose levels—good news, indeed, considering how quickly and almost painlessly the tests can now be done. But still people get it wrong. Practice in doing these tests doesn't necessarily make perfect, as we discuss shortly in

The Proof of the Pricking: Test More, Suffer Less

Can frequent glucose testing really pay off?

Researchers themselves needed to be convinced, so back in 1983 they embarked on a 10-year study to find out. Conducted by the National Institute of Diabetes and Digestive and Kidney Diseases (NID-DKD), the study divided 1,441 people with type 1 diabetes into two groups, one of which monitored their glucose levels on a standard schedule of two or three times daily, the other on a more intensive regimen of four to seven times daily. The insulin schedules of the two groups also varied. The "standard" treatment group took just two insulin injections a day, while the test group administered three or four injections based on their monitoring results. (Due to increased risks for low blood sugar [hypoglycemia] that strict glucose control can entail, such a regimen may not be advisable for the elderly or young children, for whom hypoglycemia can impose greater risks.)

"The Importance of Accuracy, and How to Get It." Keep that in mind as you review the three basic steps in glucose monitoring and where slipups can occur.

Step 1: The Prick

The first step is the pricking of a finger. (Another part of the body can be chosen—the ear lobes and toes, for example—but most people find the fingers most convenient.) Massage the hand to be tested, trying to pull blood from the palm out to the fingertips. This step should be less painful if you prick the side of your finger rather than the tip (see figure 4.2). The puncturing can be done directly with an instrument called a *lancet* or with a spring-activated unit that holds and thrusts a pricking device similar to a lancet, making the job easier for the squeamish. Another advantage of the spring-activated units is that they can be adjusted for depth of penetration.

The results of the study surprised even the researchers. The group practicing tight glucose control enjoyed the following benefits compared to the group whose control was more lax:

- 76 percent lower risk for developing eye disease (retinopathy)

- 60 percent lower risk for developing nerve disease (neuropathy)

- 50 percent lower risk for developing kidney disease (nephropathy)

- 35 percent lower risk for developing high cholesterol levels

Even though the study involved only type 1 patients, researchers feel confident that strict glucose control could produce similar benefits for people with type 2 diabetes as well.

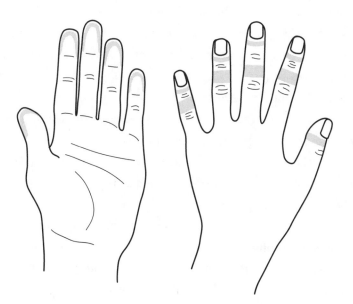

Figure 4.2—*Sites to Prick*

Step 2: The Transfer

Once you've drawn the blood, the next step is to get it to the test strip or meter that's going to be assessing its glucose content. To avoid tainting the sample with any naturally occurring oils that may be on your skin, try to allow the drop of blood to fall onto the designated test area without actually touching your finger to the testing surface. Also, if your meter is a type that requires excess blood to be wiped from the pad before testing, be sure to use only a material (such as a cotton ball or sterilized piece of gauze) recommended by the manufacturer that won't contaminate the sample or leave fibers capable of confounding the meter's results.

Step 3: The Read

This is the easy part because glucose monitoring has come a long way since the days when the only test strips available relied on the tester having to distinguish between different colors for an accurate read (see "Other Self-Testing Options," page 113). Today most test strips are designed to be read by special glucose meters, which come in many shapes, sizes, price ranges, and options for being hooked up to computerized systems for optimal data analysis. Meters also can vary from 2 minutes to just 12 seconds in how long it takes to make their glucose reads, and some meters operate without the need for test strips at all, although these models require frequent cleaning instead.

Despite their many differences, however, all meters fall into one of two basic categories with respect to how they work. One type measures glucose concentrations within a sample of blood chemically; the other measures glucose concentrations electronically. Both display their results in the same way, however: digitally on a small screen as the number of milligrams of glucose per deciliter of blood tested. Both types also are similar in their accuracy and reliability, so price, size, speed of operation, and available options should be your primary guides in selecting the best model for you. Discuss this decision with your doctor or diabetes educator to be sure you get a model that has the capabilities that are right for you. You also might want to consider purchasing two meters—one for home use and another so you can test during the day at work without having to remember to transport a single unit back and forth.

Other Self-Testing Options

Besides the new high-tech glucose meters and the fructosamine test (discussed at length later in this chapter), two less advanced methods for testing glucose levels remain available: test strips you read by eye, and test strips for measuring glucose levels in the urine. The visually read strips indicate glucose concentrations by changing color,

> *Meters are similar in their accuracy and reliability, so price, size, speed of operation, and available options should be your primary guides in selecting the best model.*

and they can be as accurate as the meter-read strips for people experienced in using them. Testing glucose levels in the urine is not generally recommended, however, for several reasons. First, glucose doesn't show up in the urine until levels in the blood are quite high. Another problem is that glucose in the urine represents what was going on in the blood several hours before—not very useful in making meaningful adjustments in medication or diet for the moment at hand. Then, too, urine testing cannot test for hypoglycemia by showing when glucose levels are low, which is often a very important reason for testing in the first place. Yet another drawback is that glucose in the urine can be altered by vitamin C, aspirin, and fluid intake. Consider testing for glucose in the urine a last resort only.

THE IMPORTANCE OF ACCURACY, AND HOW TO GET IT

As good as the new glucose meters are, they are not infallible because the people using them are not infallible. Research has shown, in fact, that while patients often demonstrate good testing techniques and get good accuracy when they finish being trained by their diabetes

The Meter Matters: Put Precision First

Prior to 1960, the only way to measure glucose levels in the blood was by way of expensive techniques that had to be done by a professional laboratory, but now small portable devices called *blood glucose meters* put the testing process conveniently and almost painlessly in the patient's hands. Devices are available even for the blind that report glucose readings by way of an electronic voice that can communicate in as many as seven different languages. Since manufacturers are upgrading their products and coming out with new models all the time, it's impossible to predict what will be available by the time you read this book, but we can give some general guidelines you should follow when faced with the purchasing process.

Accuracy should be your primary concern. In his book, *Dr. Bernstein's Diabetes Solution,* Richard K. Bernstein, M.D., who has had type 1 diabetes for more than 50 years, recommends buying only from a supplier who will refund your money if the unit you purchase fails to satisfy this accuracy requirement. To determine the accuracy prior to purchase, Dr. Bernstein recommends giving the device a trial run in the store before closing the deal. Ask permission

educators, the accuracy of their testing tends to decrease over time. People tend to get lazy about paying the amount of attention accurate testing requires. And an inaccurate result may be even more dangerous than no testing at all if results are misleadingly off the mark. The following areas are where inaccuracies most commonly tend to occur:

- **Insufficient or contaminated blood**. For glucose meters to perform as they're designed, they need an adequate amount of blood to test, and the blood needs to be free of any potentially confounding contaminants. To assure a pure and adequate sample, remember to follow the guidelines we described earlier

to perform five tests with the device, in succession, and buy it only if all five results vary by no more than 5 percent. You also can request to do a similar evaluation with sample units supplied by your physician or diabetes educator.

Here are some other factors to consider in selecting your meter:

- Is the unit compatible with the computer program your doctor may want to use to evaluate its results?

- Is the unit one that will be paid for by your health insurance?

- Does the unit give results quickly enough for you? Some can produce results in as little as 12 seconds, while others can take as long as 2 minutes.

- Is the device easy enough to use? Some are so tiny that a lot of manual dexterity is required.

- Does the device have a memory system so that results can be evaluated over an extended period?

- Are the test strips used by the meter reasonable in cost?

- Are the batteries used by the device easy enough to get and not prohibitively expensive?

in "Step 2: The Transfer." Wash your hands before testing, and allow the blood to drop onto the test strip instead of rubbing it on with your finger directly.

- **Old or uncalibrated test strips**. The test strips used by your meter must be fresh. If exposed to air, they can deteriorate in just a few hours. Always be sure to check the expiration date on unopened strips, too. Also remember that with each new batch of test strips, you may need to recalibrate your meter to use them properly if your meter is not a type that does this automatically. (No two batches of strips are exactly alike.)

- **An unmonitored meter**. Your meter itself should be tested regularly to assure that it's operating with optimal accuracy. Most models will come with a special test solution and instructions for doing this, so be sure to check the operating manual closely. You also may need to clean your meter regularly, so review the owner's instructions for this, too.

- **Faulty technique**. All the prior bases could be covered, but you still could be getting inaccurate test results if there's a problem with your testing technique. If you're using a glucose meter, be sure you're using it precisely according to the instructions as specified by its manufacturer. Pay particular attention to producing an adequate blood sample and spreading it completely over the test strip as indicated. It also can be a good idea to have your technique evaluated by a member of your health care team by performing a test in their presence to see if they might pick up something you're doing wrong. Also ask your doctor whether you can do an accuracy evaluation of your testing techniques—and also your testing equipment—by comparing the results of a test you do with your own equipment with the results of a test done on the same occasion by your doctor that is processed by your doctor's laboratory. (Be sure to do a fasting glucose test, however, because after eating, blood can show higher glucose if taken from the finger as compared to blood taken from a vein, as your doctor's test probably will do.)

- **A faulty meter**. If the results of the test you do yourself differ from those done by the lab by more than 15 percent, your final step is to check with your device's manufacturer to see whether the problem may lie with your meter. Ask for a replacement, and repeat the lab comparison test until you get a satisfactory result. Accuracy is everything with glucose testing, remember, so be persistent in doing everything you can in order to get it.

Should you expect perfection in your self-testing efforts? No. Even when testing is highly accurate and frequent, it's impossible for a person with diabetes to control blood sugar levels as delicately as the body is able to do without the disease. The body's system of checks and balances that cues the pancreas to produce just the right amount of insulin at just the right times is so sophisticated that it would be impossible to duplicate even if glucose monitoring were done every minute of every day.

This is no reason to scrimp on your monitoring efforts, however. As mentioned, research now leaves no doubt that the ill effects of diabetes can be minimized in direct proportion to how well glucose levels are kept within a normal range—and diligent glucose monitoring is the key to doing just that.

DOCTOR-ASSISTED AND OTHER TESTS: MORE TOOLS FOR DIABETES MASTERY

Self-testing for glucose levels several times daily is invaluable for helping control diabetes, but such monitoring can be even more valuable when combined with other kinds of tests. Some are performed by a member of your health care team; some you can do yourself.

To See the Bigger Picture: Testing for Hemoglobin A1c

Daily glucose monitoring is great for telling you how your blood sugar levels are doing at any given moment, but it is not as valuable for letting you know the average performance of your blood sugar levels over extended periods. This is because glucose levels can change as often as every 5 minutes. While you might catch levels that are low several times in a row, these readings would not reflect periods between those tests when your levels could have been very high.

One type of test, called the *hemoglobin A1c*, gives a truer picture by indicating how blood sugar levels are behaving over longer periods.

The test is done by your doctor, and it should be performed approximately every 3 months for people with type 1 diabetes and people with type 2 taking insulin, and every 6 months for people with type 2 not taking insulin.

The test works by measuring a component in the blood called *glycohemoglobin* that acts as a kind of sponge, picking up molecules of glucose slowly but predictably over periods of as long as 3 months. The more glucose found to be attached to this glycohemoglobin when the test is given, therefore, the more total amount of glucose has been present in the blood during the period in question.

> *The hemoglobin A1c gives a truer picture by indicating how blood sugar levels are behaving over longer periods.*

According to the latest research, the average hemoglobin A1c in the United States for people with type 2 diabetes is about 9.4 percent, which corresponds to an average glucose level of about 220 milligrams/deciliter. The ADA currently recommends taking action to control blood glucose if the hemoglobin A1c is 8 percent or greater, with the goal being less than 7 percent.

Unfortunately, not all labs report hemoglobin A1c tests in the same way. That situation could be changing shortly, however, as efforts are underway to have results standardized according to just one system.

The Home Fructosamine Test

This method of glucose monitoring could be done only by professional laboratories until 1997, when the federal Food and Drug Administration approved a do-it-yourself system for use at home. The test is similar to the hemoglobin A1c test in that it measures glucose bound to protein in the blood, but it differs in that it gives readings based on the previous 2 to 3 weeks of metabolic activity as compared to the A1c's 2 to 3 months. This faster turnover makes fructosamine tests useful for assessing the effectiveness of changes in treatment, such as switches in medication or other treatment protocols, and the tests can serve a purpose for people who otherwise would not test themselves at all. They should not, however, be used in place of daily monitorings or hemoglobin A1c tests done by your doctor.

Testing for Ketones

Besides regular testing for glucose, people with type 1 diabetes should test for ketones, harmful compounds produced when the body must resort to burning fat instead of glucose for energy. We met these compounds in chapter 1, and as a quick reminder, they can lead to serious complications including coma and even death if allowed to reach high levels. They should be tested for any time glucose levels are found to be 240 milligrams/deciliter or higher; during illness (and especially if the illness is accompanied by vomiting or diarrhea); during periods of acute stress; following a major surgery; or whenever certain symptoms appear, including mental confusion, difficulty breathing, stomach pains, or sweet, fruity-smelling breath. These could be signs of dangerously high concentrations of ketones in the blood, called ketoacidosis. As the body tries to rid itself of these harmful by-products, they collect in the urine, where they can be detected quickly and easily using a test designed for home use.

The test is done by inserting ketone-sensitive strips (available from your physician or a medical supply store) into a sample of urine. The strips are designed to change color depending on the concentration of ketones they encounter. The

> *K*etones collect in the urine, where they can be detected quickly and easily using a test designed for home use.

darker the color (usually purple), the greater the ketone concentration, and the more serious the situation. You should call your doctor's office right away if you discover higher than normal levels. You may be instructed to treat yourself with more than your usual amount of insulin. In addition, it can be helpful to drink lots of water to help dilute ketone concentrations in the blood. The most important thing is to call your doctor right away, because he or she may have more specific advice given your particular condition. Do *not* assume the condition will simply resolve on its own. An estimated 75,000 people every year are hospitalized for ketoacidosis, and 4,000 die of the condition.

Other Tests to Keep You Healthy: Stopping Trouble Before It Starts

The blood may be where diabetes begins, but some other vital parts of the body are where the disease eventually can do its most serious damage. Certain tests are now available, however, that usually can prevent such problems by detecting signs of their development before serious harm has been done. Some of these tests should be done each time you visit your doctor, others just once a year. Do consider them an important part of your treatment program, however—the key to stopping trouble before it starts.

*D*o not *assume a higher than normal ketone level will simply resolve on its own.*

For Healthy Kidneys

The kidneys are highly susceptible to being damaged by diabetes because their job is to filter the blood—not an easy job when the blood is made thick and adhesive with excess glucose. The heavy concentrations, in time, can begin to damage the delicate filtering devices in the kidneys called the *glomeruli*, and eventually the kidneys can cease functioning entirely, leading to death unless the blood is filtered mechanically by dialysis. The kidneys can be protected, however, if damage is detected early by testing for a protein in the urine called *microalbuminuria*. The test should be done as soon as possible after type 2 diabetes is first diagnosed, and within 5 years after type 1 is first found. Even if the test produces negative results, it should be repeated every year because kidney damage is preventable if caught in its earliest stages. In addition to bringing glucose under the tightest control possible and guarding against excess cholesterol and triglyc-erides in the blood, treatment may include a drug called an ACE in-hibitor until proper kidney function is restored.

To Keep Vision Clear

The eyes also are highly vulnerable to damage from diabetes because high blood sugar levels can harm both the tiny blood vessels of the eyes in addition to many of the delicate membranes making up the lens and retina. Because damage is progressive and usually develops slowly, however, serious complications usually can be avoided if prob-lems are discovered early and glucose levels are strictly controlled. Even complications that are fairly well established often can be success-fully treated with new surgical techniques, so regular eye exams should definitely be a high priority for people with type 1 and type 2 diabetes alike.

Serious eye complications usually can be avoided if problems are discovered early and glucose levels are strictly controlled.

Eye examinations should be done by an oph-thalmologist—not just an ordinary physician—every year. Even if such exams aren't part of your current treatment program, inform your doctor that they should be. Eye problems currently are among the most common complications of diabetes, but with the new advances being made in their treatment, their incidence could be reduced dramatically if people would be more diligent about having regular eye exams.

To Protect the Feet

The feet are another body part especially vulnerable to being dam-aged by the high blood sugars of poorly controlled diabetes, so they should be examined at each physician visit—at least four times a year for people who take insulin and at least twice annually for people who do not. Patients also should keep close watch for any loss of sensation or signs of infection or irritation and report any problems to their health care team right away. A device for self-testing for loss of nerve function in the feet can be obtained from the National Institutes of

Diabetes and High Blood Pressure:
An Especially Dangerous Duo

Not only can diabetes make high blood pressure more likely, high blood pressure can make diabetes more dangerous. Over 50 percent of people with diabetes over the age of 50 have high blood pressure, and when high blood pressure develops, all of the complications of diabetes are made worse. This includes damage to the kidneys, heart, blood vessels, nerves, and eyes. Controlling high blood pressure in treating diabetes is absolutely essential, therefore, and many experts feel that people with diabetes should strive for levels even lower than the standard of 135/85 considered the upper range of normal for the general population. This consensus comes based on new research showing that people with diabetes gain additional protection from complications when they maintain blood pressure levels at the low rather than high end of the normal range.

Better yet, it doesn't appear that great changes in blood pressure, even if it's relatively high, are needed to make a sizeable difference

Health by calling (800) 438-5383 and asking for the "Feet Can Last a Lifetime" package.

Basic care of the feet also is important for preventing problems, including keeping them well moisturized, avoiding undue pressure on the feet that can be caused by poorly fitting shoes, being extremely careful whenever barefoot, and not smoking. Circulation to the feet is compromised enough by diabetes without the additional constraints imposed by the noxious components of tobacco.

For a Healthy Heart

While diabetes may not cause heart disease directly, it certainly can do so indirectly by encouraging the development of three of the primary risk factors for damaging the heart. Both type 1 and type 2 dia-

in reducing diabetes risks. According to the United Kingdom Prospective Diabetes Study completed in 1998, lowering systolic blood pressure (the higher reading) by only 10 points and diastolic blood pressure by a mere 5 points resulted in a 24 percent reduction in complications while lowering death rates by 32 percent. That's a lot of reward for not a lot of work.

Yet have such findings spurred doctors to do a good job of helping patients keep their blood pressures down? Sadly, they have not. One recent study found that only about 15 percent of diabetics currently have blood pressures as low as 140/90, while only 5 percent are maintaining levels in the more preferred range of 130/85. You might consider bringing this to the attention of your health care team if your own levels are substantially higher than these levels. Your blood pressure should be checked at every visit, and measures should be taken to lower it if it's high.

betes increase risks for high blood pressure and elevated blood fats, and type 2 diabetes can increase risks for becoming overweight. These three risk factors together can make life very difficult for the heart, which may explain why more people with type 2 diabetes die of heart disease than any other complication type 2 is known to cause. To reduce their heart disease risks, people with diabetes should have their blood pressure and weight checked at every doctor visit, while blood fats should be checked at least yearly.

WORTH EVERY MINUTE

In summary, consider frequent monitoring to be your key to stopping trouble before it starts. Your goal should be to keep your blood sugar as stable as possible, remember, and only by keeping a close eye on it can you do that. Think of your blood sugar levels as being like a rambunctious two-year-old: much less apt to get into trouble if closely watched.

CHAPTER 5

New Hope for the Taste Buds

Your Cake and Glucose Control, Too

✌

HOW IMPORTANT IS diet for controlling the high blood sugars of diabetes? How important are the brakes and gas pedal to controlling your car?

Food is what produces most of your body's glucose in the first place—and some foods produce more glucose than others—so yes, what you eat can put you in the driver's seat when it comes to keeping your glucose levels under control.

Not just *what* you eat can make a difference in your blood sugar levels, however: *How much* you eat at a given sitting and *how fast* you eat also will affect how quickly and how high your blood sugar will rise. If you like to eat—and most people with type 2 diabetes do—this is not a chapter to miss, especially since it comes bearing some really great news.

Just as recent advances have given new hope in other areas of treatment, diabetes researchers have made discoveries that offer new hope in the area of diet, too: After decades of research and debate, scientists have concluded that diabetes does not have to be a death sentence for the taste buds after all. On the contrary, certain former no-no's have been found to be quite permissible—no more disruptive to glucose levels than some of the most healthful foods we can eat, in fact. This allows the refrigerator door to swing open a lot wider not just for all the gourmets with diabetes but also for those of us who would just like to enjoy a good milkshake now and again.

> *Certain former no-no's have been found to be quite permissible—no more disruptive to glucose levels than some of the most healthful foods we can eat.*

The new dietary leniency reflects not just new nutritional discoveries, moreover, but some important psychological realizations, too. "We've learned that for any diet to be effective in stabilizing blood sugar, it's got to be one that can be enjoyed, because it simply won't be followed for very long if it's not," says Liz Daily, R.N., a certified diabetes educator at the Methodist Diabetes Center in Indianapolis, Indiana. Eating is simply too basic a human pleasure to be denied, and the latest dietary guidelines from the American Diabetes Association (ADA) respect this.

So strike the word *boring* from your culinary vocabulary, grab your apron, check your spice rack, and get ready to "crank it up a notch." With a pinch of imagination and dash of know-how, you really can have your cake and glucose control, too.

A PLEASANT SURPRISE

"Guilty as charged. It was denial in the first degree. What more can I say?"

What Jackie, a 52-year-old hair stylist and owner of her own salon, is confessing here is that for 10 years she went without a medical checkup because in her heart she knew. She knew she had diabetes, but because she had seen her mother go through it, "not even being able to put sugar on her oatmeal," Jackie was just going to keep her "little secret" to herself. "If I let anyone else know, then I'd have to do something about it," she says. "So I just sat tight and hoped for the best."

But of course the worst was yet to come. One day Jackie blacked out while doing a perm, was rushed to the hospital, and her "little secret" was over. "My sugars were over 500," she recalls, "and they told me that if I hadn't gotten to the hospital as fast as I did, that perm I was doing might have been my last."

Why such dedicated denial when Jackie knew full well what she was up against? "Because I love to eat," she now says candidly. "I love to eat as much as I love life itself, so I wasn't sure if I wanted one without the other. My mother had a terrible time trying to stick to her diet, because she loved to eat, too, and I just wasn't going to live like that."

But the good news—and the point of this chapter—is that Jackie hasn't had to. She hasn't been stopping at the doughnut shop as often or marking the all-you-can-eat spaghetti nights at the firehouse on her calendar like she used to, but she's been "pleasantly surprised," she admits with a smile. "I might even enjoy eating more now because I don't take food so much for granted. I earn my treats and probably love them even more because of it."

Just as you can, too. Scientists have learned in recent years that diabetes does not have to mean a padlock on the cookie jar or even the sugar bowl, either. It just means moderation and restraint, making adjustments and checking your glucose levels if and when you do engage in a splurge. "There's actually no difference between the way someone with diabetes should eat and the way the rest of us should eat," says registered dietician and ADA spokesperson Diane Guagliani, R.D. "People with diabetes should eat a well-balanced diet from a wide variety of foods that's low in fat and supplies adequate nutrients and fiber. Anyone who's reluctant to be tested for diabetes because they're afraid of having to give up the joy of eating is making a very big mistake."

> *A*nyone who's reluctant to be tested for diabetes because they're afraid of having to give up the joy of eating is making a very big mistake.
>
> —DIANE GUAGLIANI, R.D.

SET A PLACE FOR PLEASURE

In this chapter we'll see how an effective diet for controlling blood sugar levels can be diverse, healthful, imaginative, and, above all, satisfying! So important is this element of satisfaction in the dietary treatment of diabetes, in fact, that you shouldn't be surprised if one of the first experts you're advised to see after being diagnosed is a nutritionist wanting to know your favorite foods—and not for the purpose of blacklisting them. "There's enough leeway in the dietary guidelines now that we can usually allow people—in moderation, of course—to include their greatest pleasures," says Ms. Daily.

Feel free to be totally honest with your nutritionist about your favorite foods with this in mind. By keeping your greatest loves secret—and sneaking them outside your dietary plan—you're missing out on the chance to enjoy them healthfully, Ms. Daily points out. "When accounted for in the overall scheme of the diet, patients usually can have their favorite foods—in restricted quantities, of course, but it's sure better than nothing. It's important that people do include their favorite foods, in fact, because they're going feel deprived and may not stick with their diet plans if they don't."

Foods are only "bad" when they're *not* accounted for, Ms. Daily points out, because it's these surprise treats that do the most to throw your glucose control for a loop. You might succeed in hiding your secret splurges from your nutritionist or doctor, but not from your blood sugar, and that's what counts. If there are certain foods you simply can't live without, treat them with the respect they deserve. Get them out on the table so you and your nutritionist can plan the rest of your diet and treatment around them. "Patients need to think long-term when planning their diets and try to accommodate their desires rather than ignore them," Ms. Daily says.

Just as there are no quick dietary fixes for being overweight, there are no quick dietary fixes for diabetes, so the dietary changes you agree to make should be ones you're prepared to live with every day for the rest of your life.

CONSISTENCY IS AS IMPORTANT AS CONTENT, AND NO FADS ALLOWED

But wait a minute, you might be thinking. Dieters losing weight can take days off as long as they get back on track. Can't people with diabetes do the same?

Not if you want to avoid the harm that the high blood sugar caused by those days off can do. Any time your blood sugar levels are elevated, cells in your body are suffering. Try to remember that just as important as the content of your diet is the *consistency* of your diet, because only by being consistent can you organize and implement the rest of your treatment to keep your blood sugar under the best control. Diet has been called the cornerstone of diabetes treatment for just this reason: It provides the foundation on which all other aspects of your treatment need to be based, and if that foundation is shaky, so, too, will be the entire "house." Food is what produces most of your body's glucose in the first place, remember, so the more predictable your food intake can be, the more predictable your glucose levels are going to be, and the more accurately your medication and exercise needs can be tailored to accommodate them. What you don't want to be doing is riding a dietary seesaw, being "good" one day so you can be "bad" the next. This can throw your body more curve balls than a Cy Young Award winner, guaranteeing you'll strike out in controlling your blood sugar.

> *Trying to be good one day so you can be bad the next can throw your body more curve balls than a Cy Young Award winner, guaranteeing you'll strike out in controlling your blood sugar.*

Also highly inadvisable is relying on the latest fad diet for quick weight loss to lower glucose levels, says Karmeen Kulkarni, M.S., R.D., a leading certified diabetes educator who spoke at a recent meeting of the American Medical Association to discuss recent developments in diabetes treatment and care. Yes, weight loss is an important component for treating type 2 diabetes in most cases, but not in the way these crash diets go about it, Ms. Kulkarni says.

High-protein, low-carbohydrate diets, for example, may appear to be effective at reducing weight initially, but, in fact, they only cause the body to lose large amounts of water stored in the muscles, which is easily regained. These diets also can cause drops in glucose levels, which may impress patients at first, yet generally will last only as long as the diet is followed, which for health reasons, Ms. Kulkarni says, should not be for very long. High-protein diets, most of which also are high in fat, can increase risks for heart disease and strokes, which are high enough in most people with diabetes as it is.

All things considered, the benefits in blood sugar control that may be gained by a very low-carbohydrate diet simply don't justify what it gives up in the areas of good nutrition and ease of use, most experts now agree. But if you're interested in attempting this more radical and rigorous dietary approach to blood sugar control, by all means talk to your doctor before even considering it. And if you'd like to find out more about what some experts claim this approach has to offer, check out *Dr. Bernstein's Diabetes Solution* by Richard K. Bernstein, M.D. Dr. Bernstein is himself a type 1 diabetic for whom a low-carbohydrate program combined with vigorous daily exercise has worked very well. (For more information on Dr. Bernstein's program, you can also call his clinic in Mamaroneck, New York, at [914] 698-7525.)

> *A*ny diet involving a magic or miracle food, very rapid weight loss, no exercise, bizarre quantities of food, special food combinations, or rigid menus must be held suspect.
>
> —KARMEEN KULKARNI

Nor are diets at the other end of the spectrum—low-fat, high-carbohydrate—necessarily any safer for people with diabetes, Ms. Kulkarni says. Because these diets often replace fat with sugar, they run the risk of increasing insulin resistance, which, like increased risks for heart disease and strokes, usually is a problem for most people with type 2 diabetes already. These dangers aside, "Fad diets are not founded on evidence using well-controlled, well-planned, long-term studies," Ms. Kulkarni says. "Any diet involving a magic or miracle food, very rapid weight loss, no exercise, bizarre quantities of food, special food combinations, or rigid menus must be held suspect."

EXCESS CALORIES ARE THE CULPRITS

The more researchers look at the importance of diet in treating diabetes, the more they've come to realize that what's most important, rather than trying to restrict any particular type of food or food group, is simply being careful not to eat too many calories overall. As Christine Beebe, a registered dietician and certified diabetes educator, points out, our success in lowering our fat intake in this country in recent years (from 40 percent of calories to our current average of about 34) has not succeeded in lowering our rates of obesity. It's made us fatter, in fact, because we've been eating an average of 200 more calories per day from other nonfat sources.

We need to approach blood sugar control with this same type of danger in mind: Restricting any particular food group without also restricting calories overall is not going to produce the desired results. Keep that foremost in mind as you do your dietary best to keep your glucose under control. As was pointed out at a recent meeting of experts assembled to discuss where the ADA should go with its next round of dietary guidelines, as important as *what* people with diabetes eat is *how much*. Even the seemingly most healthful diet imaginable would be unhealthful, these experts agreed, if its caloric content caused gains in weight.

> *Restricting any particular food group without also restricting calories overall is not going to produce the desired results.*

Eating too many calories can confound glucose control not just in the long run by causing weight gain, moreover; it can drive glucose levels up immediately, thus causing problems in the short-term, too. Doubling the size of a food serving, for example, doesn't just double the amount of glucose it produces—it triples or even quadruples it, studies show. Clearly this points the finger at the quantity as much as the quality of your meals in keeping your glucose levels under control.

THE GLYCEMIC INDEX QUESTION: ARE ALL CARBS EQUAL?

The issue of meal size and "quantity versus quality" emerged at the ADA meeting mentioned earlier in response to recent research suggesting that not just people with diabetes but perhaps all Americans may need to pay more attention to the quality of carbohydrate foods in their diets. The concern comes based on research ongoing since the early 1980s showing that certain carbohydrate foods—those with what's been called a high glycemic index (GI)—cause more rapid rises in blood sugar than foods with a low GI score and hence may pose risks not just for people with diabetes but also for anyone concerned about controlling weight (see table 2). The faster blood sugar rises, some scientists argue, the more insulin the body must produce. This condition, in turn, not only increases risks for diabetes by overburdening the pancreas but also encourages weight gain by triggering the body to store fat while also resulting in a faster return of hunger.

Researchers at the ADA meeting explained, however, that these fears are more theoretical than real. Based on the limited amount of research done and the relatively insignificant effects that high GI foods have actually been observed to have on real people in the real world, it was decided that the GI of carbohydrate foods should be considered a nonissue—simply not something important enough for people with diabetes (or anyone, for that matter) to worry about. In Asian cultures, for example, rates of diabetes and obesity are very low even though these people eat huge amounts of rice, which is a high GI food. Yes, high GI foods *can* be unhealthful if eaten in unhealthfully large quantities, but this is true of any food. To blame a food's GI for causing obesity or diabetes is like blaming money for causing bank robberies, it was observed. In appropriate amounts and as part of a

Table 2. Glycemic Index of Common Foods

Food	Glycemic Index
Foods with a High GI Bagel Bread, French Bread, white Dates, dried Doughnut, plain Rice, white instant Potato, baked Potatoes, French fried Potatoes, instant mashed Pretzels	More than 70
Foods with an Intermediate GI Corn, sweet Ice cream Linguine Macaroni and cheese Oatmeal, quick-cooking Peaches, canned, heavy syrup Pizza, cheese Raisins Rice, brown Soup, black bean	55 to 70
Foods with a Low GI Apple Banana Barley, pearled Bread, stone ground whole wheat Grapefruit Ice cream, low-fat Kidney beans, canned Milk, skim Oatmeal, old-fashioned Orange Peanuts Potato, sweet Rice, long-grained Spaghetti Yogurt, low-fat	Less than 55

well-balanced diet, no food should be considered off-limits for people with diabetes, these experts eventually concurred.

"The total number of calories consumed is what people with diabetes and Americans in general need to worry about, not minute differences in the way various foods affect blood sugar," says former ADA president Gerald Bernstein, M.D., on the still somewhat controversial GI issue.

Weakening the position against high GI foods even more was admission by even proponents of the GI theory that the glucose response that different foods produce can vary tremendously in people from day to day, and even the foods themselves can produce different GI levels, depending on what other foods they're eaten with and how they're prepared. Mashing, dicing, pureeing, and even just cooking certain foods can increase their GI score significantly, thus raising the very valid question of whether it's a food that's to blame for raising blood sugar levels or simply how we treat it.

> *To blame a food's glycemic index for causing obesity or diabetes is like blaming money for causing bank robberies.*

Perhaps the most valid argument of all for not becoming obsessed with the GI, most experts agree, is that some of our most healthful foods are "guilty" of being high on the GI scale. Foods such as potatoes, whole grain breads, starchy vegetables, and tropical fruits have a relatively high GI number, yet they are great sources of some of our most vital nutrients that can help reduce risks of such chronic health problems as heart disease and cancer. To restrict them would risk doing more harm than good, most experts agree.

Besides, scientists point out that the small difference in blood sugar control that avoiding high GI foods might produce is insignificant compared to the blood sugar control that can be made by pursuing more useful dietary strategies, such as controlling calories, eating on a regular schedule, and getting adequate fiber and other nutrients. We should be crunching healthful foods in healthful quantities, in other words—not essentially meaningless numbers.

So if you've been hearing news that it's important to avoid certain carbohydrate foods because they raise blood sugar dangerously faster than others, allay those fears. Yes, for athletes interested in fine-tuning their blood sugar responses to certain foods for competitive purposes, GI numbers may have some value. But for the rest of us, including people with diabetes, "There simply are other aspects of diet more important to worry about," Dr. Bernstein says. First and foremost, Dr. Bernstein and most diabetes experts agree, your dietary concerns should be to:

- Eat on as regular a schedule as possible, especially if you're taking medication.

- Avoid overeating, for purposes of controlling weight as well as avoiding surges in blood glucose that overeating can cause.

- Eat a wide variety of foods to assure nutritional balance as well as dietary enjoyment.

Tips for Curbing the "Carbo" Impact

While it's true that foods high in carbohydrates raise glucose levels in the blood higher and faster than foods high in protein or fat, there are ways to mitigate this response. Many experts, in fact, feel these strategies can help erase the alleged disadvantages of eating carbohydrate foods with a high GI number because these tactics can help substantially slow a food's glucose response:

- **Eat your carbohydrates along with protein or fat**. Because protein and fat digest more slowly than carbohydrates, they can help slow the digestion of carbohydrates when eaten together. A scoop of yogurt on a baked potato, for example, or dollop of cottage cheese on a bagel can help blunt their glucose impact and add some beneficial protein and calcium, too. (High-fat toppings such as sour cream or butter also can slow glucose-production when added to carbohydrates, but at a greater caloric expense.)

- **Eat carbohydrates high in fiber.** Like protein and fat, fiber slows the digestive process and hence can lengthen the time it takes for glucose to enter the bloodstream from a carbohydrate food. Whole grain breads will produce less of a glucose rise than breads made from refined flour, for example, and whole grain cereals such as oatmeal and shredded wheat—or high-fiber cereals such as All-Bran—will boost glucose levels less than cereals made from grains robbed of their fiber by processing.

- **Cook vegetables lightly.** Not only is this a good way to spare heat-sensitive nutrients, but also vegetables will digest more slowly if they're lightly cooked. Vegetables eaten raw, of course, will digest most slowly of all.

- **Eat carbohydrates in their most solid state.** The more liquid a carbohydrate is, the faster it will digest, so opt for carbs in their most solid form possible. Corn from the cob, for example, will produce less of a glucose surge than creamed corn from a can, and fruit eaten whole will raise blood sugar less than fruit juices. Better to chew than sip, in other words, to keep blood sugar under control. Also keep the "solid state" rule in mind when preparing foods such as potatoes, carrots, turnips, and yams, which will cause less pronounced blood sugar rise when served whole than if chopped, diced, pureed, or mashed.

- **Let beans slow the show.** The soluble fiber in beans helps them slow the glucose production of any high GI food they accompany—a good reason to serve them often as a side dish, not just when having rice.

- **Add something acidic.** Glycemic index experts report that adding highly acidic foods such as vinegar or lemon juice to starchy foods can help slow their conversion to glucose in the bloodstream. Try a few sprinkles of vinegar on french fries, for example, or include vinegar or lemon juice when making dishes such as potato salad or noodle casseroles.

- **Eat slowly**. How fast glucose enters the bloodstream depends on how fast food enters the stomach, so by eating slowly you can reduce the blood sugar impact of whatever you eat, regardless of its nutritional makeup. Eating slowly is also a good weight control strategy because it gives the stomach ample time to realize it's full, thus reducing the tendency to overeat.

> *The more liquid a carbohydrate is, the faster it will digest, so opt for carbs in their most solid form possible.*

- **Don't overeat**. By doubling the size of a portion, you don't just double its glucose output; you increase it by as much as fourfold, so realize that "less is more" for purposes of glucose control and weight control alike.

WELL-BALANCED IS BEST

There's no way around it, the majority of experts now agree: A well-rounded diet is best, especially considering the "well-rounded" strains diabetes can put on the entire body. As noted by Harvard Medical School professor and chair of the Patient Education Committee at the Joslin Diabetes Center in Boston, Richard Beaser, M.D., "The old adage 'you are what you eat' applies to all people, but it takes on special meaning for people with diabetes." Diabetes is a disease with potential for affecting virtually every major organ, remember, so it's important to be giving those organs all the nutrients they need. A diet that controls blood sugar might take care of a few trees, in other words, but in so doing it would badly neglect the forest.

According to the ADA, your diet should help:

- Control glucose levels
- Control blood fats (triglycerides and total cholesterol)

Carbohydrates: A Chemistry Lesson

If you're a bit confused by all the variations on the carbohydrate theme, don't feel bad. There are carbohydrates said to be "simple" and "complex" and "refined"—and that's before "starches" and "sugars" get thrown into the mix. What's the difference, and does it matter?

Not as much as scientists once thought. As detailed earlier in this chapter, a "shot" that is still ringing in the ears of nutritionists the world over was fired back in the early 1980s when researchers found that table sugar and a lot of other sweet treats—long thought to be the arch villains of glucose control—caused blood sugar to rise no faster than such long-assumed nutritional good guys as potatoes, rice, and even carrots. Was this good news or bad? Did it mean that our "junk" carbohydrates weren't in fact so junky or that our healthful carbohydrates weren't in fact so healthful?

The question is still debated today, with some nutritionists maintaining that carbohydrates with a high gylcemic index (GI) need to be seen as the health robbers they really are, while the majority of health experts take less of an alarmist's view. We need simply to eat a well-balanced diet, these experts believe, setting our sites on calorie control and getting enough fiber and other nutrients in our carbohydrate foods while letting the GI numbers fall as they may.

Now for the chemistry lesson. Carbohydrates are not foods but rather collections of molecules in foods—molecules consisting of

---

- Maintain a healthy weight
- Provide adequate nutrients

It should also be *fun* to eat!

Variety Through the Food Pyramid

Balanced is best and a lot kinder to the taste buds, too. To make such a diet readily accessible, the ADA recommends that people with dia-

carbon, oxygen, and hydrogen—that Mother Nature has managed to arrange in some remarkably dissimilar ways. The cellulose that goes "crunch" in a piece of celery is a carbohydrate, for example, but then so is the maple syrup we pour on our waffles.

In the seeming chaos is some order, however, because all types of carbohydrates can be put into one of two basic categories. *Complex* carbohydrates (also referred to as *starches*) are found mostly in grain products and starchy vegetables, while *simple* carbohydrates (also called *sugars*) occur mostly in fruits, milk products, and sweet-tasting vegetables such as carrots, parsnips, and peas. Very few carbohydrate foods are composed strictly of one type of carbohydrate or the other, however, but rather are a composite of the two types together.

And where might "refined" fit into the carbohydrate picture? This term refers simply to the processing that carbohydrate foods frequently undergo—the milling that removes much of the fiber from grains, for example, and the high-tech tinkerings that turn corn into corn syrup, sugar cane into sugar, and fruits into jellies and jams. Such processing usually is done to improve the taste, texture, or shelf life of the foods it alters, but frequently at the expense of valuable nutrients, which is why eating carbohydrate foods as close as possible to their natural state generally is preferred. Processing also tends to raise the GI number of a food by removing the fiber needed to slow its digestion and hence reduce its glucose impact—yet another reason "natural" tends to be best.

betes base their diets on what's known as the "food pyramid"—the same system meant to help all Americans keep their diets on a healthful track. The pyramid categorizes all foods into one of seven basic groups, and while all seven groups should be included, some groups should make up a larger portion of the diet than others. As you can see from figure 5.1, the bulk of your calories should come from carbohydrate foods such as whole grain cereals and breads, vegetables, and fruit. These foods have the ability to reduce risks of heart disease,

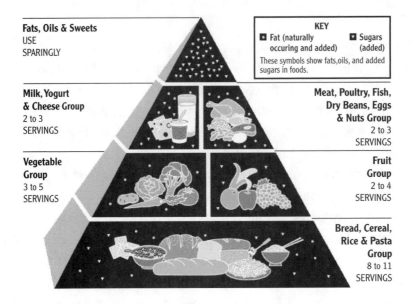

Figure 5.1—*The Food Guide Pyramid*

Source: Centers for Disease Control and Prevention

high blood pressure, and even some forms of cancer, so most experts agree they deserve to make up the bulk of the diabetic as well as general American diet.

Next on the pyramid are foods rich in protein: meat, poultry, fish, dairy products, eggs, beans, and nuts. Protein is essential for the growth and maintenance of muscle and other vital tissue, and it has the additional advantage of raising glucose levels slowly and only slightly. Protein foods that are low in fat also can be helpful for weight control because they tend to be quite filling despite being low in calories.

The foods that should be eaten most sparingly, and not just by folks with diabetes but by everyone, are fats and sweets, represented by the small triangle at the top of the pyramid. The foods in this group have the disadvantage of being essentially void of nutrients despite brimming with calories. Especially ill advised from this category are foods high in saturated fat, which has been shown to increase risks not just for heart disease, high blood pressure, and some types of cancer but insulin resistance, too. Add the obvious drawback of encouraging weight gain, and it's clear why these foods need to be kept to a minimum.

This pyramid approach to eating healthfully might seem almost childishly simple, but that's why it can work. "It doesn't demand a lot of brainwork, and people like that," says Ms. Daily, of her experience in counseling patients to eat according to the food pyramid's schematic logic. But most important, a diet based on the food

> *This pyramid approach to eating healthfully might seem almost childishly simple, but that's why it can work.*

pyramid encourages the all-important aspect of variety, which is important not just for making meals healthful but also for allowing them to be tasty, imaginative, and fun.

Seven Ways to Make the Food Pyramid Even Better

As good as the pyramid system is, however, it can be made even better. This is because not all foods within the major food groups are equal in their ability to help control diabetes, nor are they equal in their overall nutritional value. An order of French fries, for example, is not as healthful as a slice of whole grain bread, yet both technically belong to the same starch family. Nor is a strip of bacon as healthful as a serving of broiled salmon as a protein food, or a pat of butter as healthful as a teaspoon of olive oil in the fats department. Within each of the major food groups that comprise the pyramid system are some choices that are clearly better than others—and it can be worth your while to make the best choices possible. For that reason, the following guidelines are offered here to raise the value of the food pyramid—and your health—to an even higher level.

1. Select the Most Stellar Starches

What makes some foods in the starch category better choices than others? The most healthful starches are those that are low in fat and

Beans: Good for More Than Just the Heart

If one particular food could be said to stand head and shoulders above the rest in helping control the high blood sugars of diabetes, it would have to be the lowly bean. Beans have been called "gourmet preventive medicine," and this label is especially true for people with diabetes. Not only can beans reduce risks of heart attacks and stokes by helping lower cholesterol and blood pressure (important for individuals with diabetes since their risks for these mishaps can exceed those of nondiabetics by as much as fourfold), beans also can help control diabetes directly by "gumming up" the intestinal tract. As explained by University of Kentucky researcher James W. Anderson, M.D., "The soluble fiber in beans appears to 'gel' the intestinal contents, slowing the passage of glucose from food into the cells. As a result, less insulin is needed to control blood sugar, enabling some patients to discontinue their medications."

In addition to this gelling effect, beans contain an enzyme that also helps impede starch digestion. The end result is that beans can substantially slow blood sugar increases when eaten with other high-carbohydrate foods. Eating beans with rice, for example, will cause less of a blood sugar response than if the rice were eaten

high in fiber. The fiber content of a starchy food is important because more fiber means slower digestion, and hence a slower release of glucose into the bloodstream, while less fat means fewer calories, which is helpful for weight control. Try to eat more of the foods listed here with this high-fiber, low-fat goal in mind. Not only are these the best starches for controlling blood sugar in people with diabetes already diagnosed, but two recent studies by researchers from Harvard (the Nurses Health Study and the Health Professionals Follow-Up Study) have found that a diet that includes a lot of cereal fibers (a type of

alone, and adding beans to a pasta dish will slow the glucose rise caused by that starchy meal.

But beans can do more than just "put the brakes" on carbohydrate digestion; they can serve up a bushel of great nutrients, too—calcium, iron, potassium, phosphorus, magnesium, B vitamins, and zinc. Especially noteworthy because of the increased risks for heart disease that diabetes poses, beans are one of our very best sources of folate, a nutrient that recent studies show can reduce risks of heart attacks and strokes. As an added bonus, some research also shows beans can be helpful for weight control by helping blunt insulin production, thus prolonging the amount of time before hunger returns when beans are included in a meal.

All things considered, it's hard to believe such miraculous "medicine" can be had for just pennies a pound. If certain intestinal disadvantages deter you from eating more beans, know that you can silence much of their gas production by soaking them for several hours in water or by accompanying their ingestion with a few capsules of a product called Beano, which deactivates their gas-making compounds before trouble can strike. Most health food stores and pharmacies carry this helpful digestive aid.

fiber many of these foods contain) may help reduce risks for developing type 2 diabetes in the first place.

Breads: Whole wheat, multigrain, oatmeal, pumpernickel, and rye.

Cereals: Oatmeal, wheat germ, shredded wheat, and cereals designated as "high-fiber."

Grains: Brown rice, wild rice, basmati rice, bulgur, and barley.

Beans: All types, including kidney, pinto, lima, soy, navy, garbanzo, split peas, and lentils.

Pasta: Made from whole wheat or soy flour.

Potatoes: Baked or boiled rather than mashed or fried.

2. Pick the Purest Proteins

While some protein foods are, in fact, mostly protein—tuna, for example, is about 86 percent protein—many "protein" foods contain surprisingly little. A hot dog, for example, is not 86 percent protein but rather about 86 percent fat—most of it saturated fat, moreover, the kind people with diabetes need to avoid most. Many other commonly considered "protein" foods are nearly as guilty. Protein foods can come loaded with sodium and cholesterol, too, so it's worth it to make the proteins in your diet the purest proteins you can. Here are some sound selections.

> **Proteins that are lean, not "mean":** Fish and shellfish, chicken and turkey without skin, lean cuts of beef and pork with all visible fat removed, non- or low-fat dairy products, egg whites, tofu, beans.

3. Venerate, Don't Violate, Your Vegetables

Vegetables are especially important for people with diabetes because in addition to being low in calories and great sources of glucose-blunting fiber, they're our best source of nutrients known as antioxidants, which some research suggests may help protect against the long-term tissue damage diabetes can cause. To get the full benefit of these nutrients, however, be careful not to overcook vegetables (light steaming is best), and resist the urge to nullify their low-calorie advantage by smothering them in butter or a high-fat sauce. Season them, if you must, with lemon or lime juice, a light dressing, a flavored vinegar, or some fresh herbs.

> **Most viable vegetables:** Asparagus, broccoli, brussels sprouts, carrots, cauliflower, collard greens, kale, green and red peppers, squash (winter), tomatoes, turnip greens.

The Whole Truth About Whole Grain Bread

The best breads to eat to limit blood sugar surges are those made from whole grains rather than breads made from flour that has had its fiber removed through milling. Distinguishing these more healthful breads from the rest of the pack can be a little tricky, however. A bread whose label says it's "whole wheat" may simply be a bread that has been made "wholly"—meaning entirely—from wheat flour, but wheat flour that has been milled and therefore stripped of its all-important fiber.

To get around this, look to the nutritional label and check the bread's fiber content. If the bread is truly made from whole wheat flour not robbed of its bran, it should have at least 2 grams of fiber per serving. Its label also should include terms such as "100% whole wheat" or "whole grain" or "stone ground." If these terms do not appear, however, and the first ingredient listed is enriched wheat flour, the product is essentially white bread. And don't be fooled by a bread's brownish color. That, unfortunately, often comes from the addition of molasses to give it a more wholesome-looking hue.

And what about the "lite" breads that boast added fiber? They're fine. They might not be especially tasty because their fiber often comes from added vegetable fibers such as cellulose rather than wheat bran, but they're certainly preferable to white bread that typically has no appreciable fiber at all.

4. Go for the Freshest Fruit

Like vegetables, fruits are virtually fat-free, high in fiber, and loaded with vital nutrients—especially those all-important antioxidants that can help prevent tissue breakdown. Fruit also can make a healthful substitute for a more fattening goody to satisfy a craving for sweets. To get the full benefit of fruit, however, try to eat it fresh rather than canned, and whole rather than juiced. Canning often adds sugar, and juicing robs fruit of most of its fiber. All fruits have substantial nutritional value, but here are those that can be especially "fruitful" for their fiber, vitamin, and mineral content.

Most fruitful fruits: Apples, bananas, blackberries, blueberries, grapefruit, cantaloupe, oranges, peaches, pears, strawberries, watermelon.

5. Opt for the Friendliest Fats

While it's true that saturated fat—the kind prevalent in animal foods such as meat, eggs, butter, and other dairy products—can increase risks of heart disease and even some forms of cancer, other types of fat—in moderation, of course—can be downright friendly. Polyunsaturated fats, for example, found in vegetable oils such as corn, soybean, sunflower, and safflower, may actually help reduce risks of heart disease by helping to lower levels of total (LDL as well as HDL) cholesterol in the blood. And monounsaturated fats, prevalent in olive oil, canola oil, and most nuts and seeds, may be even more healthful by helping lower only LDL cholesterol (the "bad" kind) while actually giving HDL cholesterol (the "good" kind) a modest boost. New research suggests that monounsaturated fats may actually help people with diabetes control their blood sugar as well.

> *New research suggests that monounsaturated fats may actually help people with diabetes control their blood sugar as well.*

Also encouragingly healthful are the *omega-3 fatty acids* found in cold water and fatty fish such as salmon, mackerel, sardines, tuna, halibut, and cod. This type of fat has been found to reduce risks of heart attacks by helping lower fats in the blood (triglycerides), decreasing blood pressure, and also reducing the tendency of the blood to form potentially heart-stopping clots.

Friendliest fats: Monounsaturated fats (including olive oil, canola oil, peanut oil, avocados, seeds, and nuts) and polyunsaturated fats (including corn oil, sunflower oil, safflower oil and soybean oil).

Least friendly fats: Saturated fats (including butter, lard, and coconut oil) and hydrogenated fats (prevalent in most vegetable shortenings and stick margarine; whipped and "diet" margarines generally contain less).

6. Do Dairy, but Without the Fat

Dairy products are important for their calcium—your best bet for avoiding the thinning of the bones known as *osteoporosis*—but many dairy products can offer pitfalls of their own by being high in saturated fat. Whole milk and yogurt derive almost half their calories from saturated fat, for example, and most hard cheeses are at least 70 percent saturated fat. Whether it's milk, yogurt, cheese, or even a splurge of ice cream, therefore, do yourself the favor of opting for non- or low-fat varieties. Most have just as much calcium and protein as their fuller-fat kin, and give up very little in flavor. As the list here also shows, there are some very good nondairy sources of calcium, so try to include these in your diet, too.

Best low-fat dairy sources of calcium: Skim and low-fat milk, nonfat and low-fat yogurt, nonfat and low-fat cheeses.

Best nondairy sources of calcium: Sardines, shrimp, salmon, rhubarb, spinach, turnip greens, broccoli.

7. Don't Be Swindled by "Natural" or "Sugar-Free"

Yes, scientists have found that pure table sugar—sucrose—raises levels of glucose in the blood no faster than the starch in a piece of white bread (discussed earlier), but this increase is still a lot, too much to allow sucrose to be consumed in large quantities, especially since sucrose provides no nutrients and can raise levels of triglycerides in the blood in addition to raising glucose. But be aware that this goes for certain other forms of sugar, too, as the list in this section shows. Honey, for example, although "all natural," still causes the same blood sugar hikes as table sugar, as do corn syrup, molasses, and other foods commonly used in sugar's stead.

Bad. These sweeteners can have the same effect as table sugar (sucrose) in raising levels of glucose in the blood, so keep an eye out for them on nutritional labels: carob, corn syrup, dextrin, dextrose, honey, lactose, maltodextrin, maltose, molasses, saccharose, sorghum.

Better. These sweeteners do not raise glucose levels as much as table sugar but will produce a measurable effect, nonetheless: fructose, mannitol, sorbitol, xylitol.

Best. These sweeteners do not affect glucose levels to any appreciable degree: aspartame (Nutrasweet and Equal), saccharin (Sweet'n Low), acesulfame potassium (Sweet One), and stevia (an herbal sweetener sold in health food stores).

Nor are all sweeteners advertised as "sugar-free" necessarily permissible in unlimited amounts because many of these have calories and can raise blood sugar levels, too. Products in the "better" group such as sorbitol and xylitol might not raise glucose levels as much as table sugar and other sweeteners in the "bad" group, but they will have an effect. The only sugar-free sweetening agents that have no appreciable effect on glucose levels are those in the "best" group, so pay attention when selecting foods advertised as sugar-free with this in mind. Sugar-free does not necessarily mean trouble-free when it comes to how much a product will raise glucose levels in the blood.

> *Sugar-free does not necessarily mean trouble-free when it comes to how much a product will raise glucose levels in the blood.*

Size Matters

The food pyramid, as you have seen, recommends numbers of servings from each of the major food groups. But what constitutes a serving? A lineman for the Denver Broncos could certainly be expected to have a different idea than a senior citizen. It's important that you learn what a serving really does constitute, however, because the quantity of what you eat is as important for controlling blood sugar as the quality. The most healthful diet in the world is *not* going to be healthful if you eat too much of it. Try to stick to the following serving sizes with that in mind:

- **The grain group**. A serving is considered to be one slice of bread, one half of a hamburger bun or English muffin, three to four large crackers, or 1/2 cup of cereal, rice, or pasta (an amount about the size of a scoop of ice cream).

- **The vegetable group**. A serving here is 1/2 cup of chopped or cooked vegetables, or 1 cup of leafy vegetables such as spinach or kale.

- **The fruit group**. A serving is 1/2 cup of fruit that is chopped or cooked or a medium-sized piece of fruit (about the size of a tennis ball) if eaten whole.

- **The dairy group**. Consider a serving to be 1 cup of milk, 11/2 ounces of natural cheese, or 2 ounces of processed cheese (an ounce of cheese is about the size of four dice).

- **The protein group**. A serving is one egg, 1/2 cup of cooked beans, or 2 to 3 ounces of meat, poultry, or fish (a portion about the size of a deck of playing cards).

FAST FOODS: KNOW YOUR FRIENDS FROM YOUR FOES

They're convenient, fast, affordable, and everywhere. But are fast-food restaurants emporiums of glucose chaos for people with diabetes?

Possibly as much as for any other question ever asked, that depends. You can consume more calories and fat in a single fast-food meal than you should eat in an entire day, or you can order a meal as healthful as any you could make at home even with your nutritionist watching over your shoulder. For example, a Double Whopper from Burger King

with a large order of fries and a large soda tips the scales at 2,000 calories and 85 grams of fat. Also available at Burger King, however, is a
broiled chicken sandwich that, if you hold the mayo and order a sugar-
free soda, comes in at 370 calories and only 9 grams of fat.

The key to navigating your way healthfully through the likes of
the Golden Arches is to get to know the menus and "have it your
way" by ordering items without their high-fat sauces or dressings
whenever possible. The mayonnaise or similar "secret sauce" on most
chicken sandwiches, for example, is worth about 150 calories and 15
grams of fat with virtually no nutrients to show for it. Here are some
other basic calorie-saving pointers to keep in mind the next time you
find yourself about to speak into that drive-through microphone:

- **Steer clear of deep-fried.** Along with the breaded coating,
  deep-frying easily can add more than 100 calories to an entrée—
  and most of them from fat. While a breaded and fried chicken
  sandwich from Hardee's offers 480 calories and 18 grams of fat,
  for example, that same sandwich made with grilled chicken
  checks in at only about 350 calories and 11 grams of fat.

- **Know that "large" means exactly that.** A big part of the problem with fast food isn't always its quality as much as its quantity.
  Does a soda really have to be as large as a quart of milk (32
  ounces), and do we really need *two* all-beef patties rather than
  just one? Not unless we want our waistlines coming in a "large,"
  too, and our blood sugar soaring out of control. Opt for "small"
  whether ordering a burger, fries, pizza, or a shake.

- **Go for the entrées with the fewest adjectives**. An item advertised simply as a "hamburger" is going to have fewer calories
  and less fat than something offered as "super," "supreme,"
  "royale," or "deluxe." The leaner the descriptive language,
  generally speaking, the leaner the product.

- **Beware of the high-fat "booby traps."** These are items with
  names that sound healthful but get you with hidden or added

fat. A "Taco Salad" at Taco Bell, for example, serves up a monstrous 800 calories and 50 grams of fat, thanks largely to its avalanche of high-fat dressing. Order such calorie-laden condiments on the side whenever possible.

- **Know your toppings.** Whether you're adorning a pizza or a hamburger, know that toppings such as cheese, bacon, and sausage are going to add a lot more fat and calories than vegetable selections such as onions, mushrooms, peppers, and tomatoes. You get a lot more fiber and other healthful nutrients in the vegetable toppings, too.

- **If in doubt, ask for the nutritional facts.** Most fast-food restaurants now have nutritional fact sheets on all the items they sell, but you'll need to request this information at the counter—*before* you place your order.

Best Fast-Food Choices

Not all fast foods have to smother you with their calories and fat. Here's a rundown of fast-food offerings that have fewer than 400 calories and also—to keep the American Diabetes and American Heart Associations happy—serve up less than 30 percent of their calories from fat (see table 3). And please trust that all the items offered by these restaurants were given a chance to qualify for the list; what you see here are the only ones that made the grade. Many foods offered at these eateries have well over 600 calories with over 60 percent fat of their calories coming from fat, proving just how important it is to know your fast-food friends from your foes.

EATING OUT: YOUR HEALTH AND "HAUTE" CUISINE, TOO

Dining out at a fine restaurant is one of life's greatest pleasures, and there's no reason diabetes should get in its way. There are some basic

Table 3. Fast-Food Choices with Low Calorie and Fat Content

Restaurant	Food	Calories	Fat (grams)
Arby's	Roast beef sandwich	296	10
	Roast chicken sandwich	276	6
	Roast turkey sandwich	260	7
	Grilled BBQ sandwich	388	13
	Baked potato, plain	355	3
Burger King	BK Broiler chicken sandwich, without mayo	370	9
	Milkshake, small vanilla or chocolate	330	7
Chick-fil-A	Hearty chicken soup	110	1
	Char-grilled chicken garden salad	170	3
	Chicken salad plate	290	5
	Chick-n-strips salad	290	9
	Chick-fil-A sandwich	290	9
	Chick-fil-A chicken salad sandwich on whole wheat	320	5
	Chick-fil-A chargrilled chicken sandwich	280	3
	Icedream, small cone	140	4
Hardee's	Grilled chicken sandwich	359	11
	Grilled chicken salad	150	3
	Baked beans, 5 ounces	170	1
	Mashed potatoes, 4 ounces	70	1
	Ice cream cone	170	2
	Milkshake, small vanilla or chocolate	350	5

(continues)

Kentucky Fried Chicken (KFC)	Chicken breast, tender roast without skin	169	4.5
	Chicken sandwich, barbecue-flavored	265	8
	Baked beans	190	3
	Corn on the cob	150	1.5
McDonald's	Bagel, plain	310	1
	Apple-bran muffin, low-fat	300	3
	Grilled chicken sandwich, without mayo	300	5
	Grilled chicken salad	120	1.5
	Milkshake, small vanilla or chocolate	360	9
	Ice cream cone, vanilla	150	2.5
Pizza Hut (figures based on one piece of a medium pie)	Edge, chicken/veggie	120	3
	Edge, veggies	110	2.5
	Edge, The Works	140	5
	Hand tossed, Chicken Supreme	240	6
	Hand tossed, ham	230	6
	Hand tossed, Veggie Lover's	240	7
	Thin 'N Crispy, ham	190	6
	Thin 'N Crispy, Veggie Lover's	170	6
Subway (6-inch sandwich, wheat roll)	Ham	302	5
	Roast beef	303	5
	Roast chicken	348	6
	Turkey	289	5
	Turkey and ham	295	5
	Veggie Delight	237	3
Taco Bell	Burrito, bean	380	12
	Burrito, grilled chicken	400	14
	Taco, soft, grilled chicken	200	6

Source: Adapted from *The Complete Book of Food Counts* by Corinne T. Netzer (Dell, 2000)

guidelines you should follow; however, to help make your experience as healthful as possible:

- **Call ahead**. It can be helpful to know in advance whether the restaurant is willing to accommodate special requests.

- **Be inquisitive**. If you're unsure of what ingredients are in a particular dish, don't be afraid to ask.

- **Be bold**. If you don't feel comfortable with a particular dish, ask if it can be altered to suit you.

- **Be consistent**. Try to eat portions similar to what you'd eat at home, and don't be afraid to ask for a doggie bag for leftovers.

- **Be forceful**. If a dish normally is served with a sauce or gravy that may be too high in fat or calories, ask that it be omitted or served on the side. The same applies to method of preparation: If a dish is normally served deep-fried or sautéed in a lot of butter, ask if it might be poached or broiled "dry," instead, to reduce fat and caloric content.

- **Learn the lingo**. At some upscale restaurants, the menu may be a little difficult to decipher, especially if it's French in origin. Here's a quick vocabulary lesson to help you make sense of some of the loftier culinary jargon you may encounter.

ail—garlic
au gratin—with cheese
beurre—butter
boeuf—beef
bouille—boiled
canard—duck
champignons—mushrooms
crème—cream
farci—stuffed
frit—fried

gratiné—baked in a coating of bread crumbs
grille—broiled
jambon—ham
legumes—vegetables
mousse—thickened with cream
nouilles—noodles
oeufs—eggs
pane—breaded
poche—poached

pommes de terre—potatoes

porc—pork

poulet—chicken

riz—rice

salade—salad

sauté—pan-fried in butter

veau—veal

vin—wine

HOW HEALTHFUL IS YOUR DIET?

Your diet is important not just for helping to keep your blood sugar under control but for keeping you strong and healthy for combating potential complications of diabetes, too. How good a job is your current diet doing at achieving this dual goal? This following quiz can help you find out. Good luck, and if you do poorly, don't despair. Just think of how much better you're going to feel when you do get it in shape.

1. At which of these meals would you say you generally consume the most calories?
    a) breakfast
    b) lunch
    c) dinner
    d) bedtime snack

2. How often do you skip meals?
    a) never
    b) a few times a month
    c) a few times a week
    d) you've already skipped one today

3. Are you generally one to try the latest fad diet to lose weight?
    a) absolutely not
    b) you've tried one or two in your life
    c) you've tried perhaps a half dozen in your life
    d) you've lost count and are actually on one right now

4. In an average day, how many servings of vegetables would
   you say you eat?
   a) five or more
   b) two to four
   c) fewer than two
   d) French fries are generally as close as you get

5. In an average day, how many servings of fruit (fresh, frozen,
   or canned) would you say you eat?
   a) four or more
   b) two or three
   c) fewer than three
   d) usually none, unless strawberry ice cream counts

6. Which of the following best describes your customary way of
   eating potatoes?
   a) baked, with low-fat yogurt instead of butter or sour cream
      as a topping
   b) baked with butter or sour cream
   c) mashed, with butter
   d) French fried, preferably with melted cheese

7. Which of the following is the type of milk you most often
   drink?
   a) skim
   b) 1 or 2 percent fat
   c) whole
   d) chocolate

8. Which of the following would you say are your primary
   sources of protein?
   a) beans and other vegetable proteins
   b) skinless poultry and/or fish
   c) beef and pork
   d) fast-food entrées such as hamburgers, hot dogs, pizza, and
      fried chicken

9. What type of cereal do you most commonly eat?
   a) a high-fiber cereal such as All-Bran, or a whole grain, cooked cereal such as oatmeal, Wheateena, or Cream of Wheat
   b) a processed cereal high in vitamins such as Total or Product 19
   c) a processed cereal with a moderate vitamin content such as Cheerios, Rice Krispies, or corn flakes
   d) a processed cereal that's nice and sweet, such as Count Chocula or Fruit Loops

10. As a between-meal snack, which of the following would you think of having first?
    a) a piece of fresh fruit or maybe some celery sticks and peanut butter
    b) pretzels or air-popped popcorn
    c) cheese and crackers
    d) a candy bar

11. At a cocktail party, which of the following hors d'oeuvres would get most of your attention?
    a) crudités (raw vegetables)
    b) smoked salmon
    c) cheese and crackers
    d) little hot dogs wrapped in bacon

12. How often will you treat yourself to a really decadent dessert?
    a) a few times a month, maybe less
    b) about once a week
    c) several times a week
    d) you're feeling in the mood for a decadent dessert right now

Scoring

Give yourself 4 points for every *a* answer, 3 for every *b*, 2 for every *c*, and 1 for each *d*.

(continues)

40 to 48. Congratulations! It sounds as though you're giving your body the good nutrition it requires.

30 to 39. Not bad, but you could do better.

20 to 29. Careful—your shoddy diet could be exacerbating your diabetes as well as inviting other health problems.

19 or less. Holy Cheez Wiz! Your body deserves much better, especially to combat the physical strains imposed by diabetes.

THE (MODERATE) PLACE FOR ALCOHOL

How permissible is a "beverage of one's choice" when trying to control diabetes?

That depends on the beverage and how often it's chosen. Moderate consumption of alcohol—defined as no more than one drink a day for women and two a day for men—usually is permissible if glucose is under good control. Because alcohol contains a lot of calories, however—7 per gram, or almost twice as many as carbohydrates and only two fewer than fats—these calories must be taken into consideration for purposes of weight control. Because many sweet-tasting alcoholic beverages also contain a lot of carbohydrates in the form of sugar (see table 4) these also must be acknowledged if such beverages are to be a part of your dietary plan. Here are some other important considerations you should be aware of if you intend to include alcoholic beverages in your diet:

- Alcohol can magnify the effects of insulin, thus increasing risks of low blood sugar (hypoglycemia), especially if consumed on an empty stomach. People taking sulfonylureas or insulin, therefore, should drink alcohol with meals only.

- Alcohol also can increase risks of low blood sugar by inhibiting the glucose-producing ability of the liver, an effect that can last as long as 8 to 12 hours, and hence should be kept in mind the morning after. It may be especially important to eat an early and substantial breakfast.

- The effects of alcohol in lowering blood sugar can be especially pronounced following exercise—something for fun-loving fitness buffs to keep in mind when tempted to celebrate an especially good workout.

- Alcohol can impair judgment, thus increasing risks not just of dietary indiscretion but also laxity in glucose monitoring and other aspects of treatment.

- Alcohol should not be used by anyone suffering from gestational diabetes (diabetes during pregnancy), high trigylceride levels, pancreatitis, digestive problems, neuropathy (loss of nerve function), kidney disease, or certain types of heart problems. (Be sure to check with your doctor if you suspect any of these conditions may apply to you.)

- Alcohol can impair the action of some medications— diabetes medications included.

PROOF OF THE PUDDING

Can such simple lifestyle changes as diet and exercise (which we'll be examining in chapter 6) really make a difference in deterring type 2 diabetes, a disease many people fear will run its course no matter what? It's certainly something we all have a right to know before investing the kind of "elbow grease" that doctors now advise.

A study done in Finland recently set out to answer that all-important question, and the answer—reported at the American Diabetes Association's 60th Annual Scientific Sessions held in 2000, in San Antonio, Texas, was a resounding yes. The study divided 523 people (average age 55) who were in the beginning stages of developing diabetes and also were overweight into two groups—one of which was subjected to intensive counseling on the appropriate dietary and exercise changes

Table 4. Alcoholic Beverages: Know What's Going Down the Hatch

Beverage	Serving Size (ounces)	Calories	Alcohol (grams)	Carbohydrates (grams)
Beer				
Regular	12	150	13	13
Light	12	100	11	5
Distilled Spirits				
80 proof (blended whiskey, bourbon, gin, rum, scotch, vodka)	1.5	100	14	trace
Cognac, dry brandy	1	75	11	trace
Wines				
Dry white	4	80	11	trace
Red or rosé	4	85	12	trace
Sweet	4	105	12	5
Sherry, dry	4	150	18	4
Sherry, sweet	4	180	18	14
Port	4	180	18	14
Muscatel	4	180	18	14
Champagne	4	100	12	4
Cordials and liqueurs				
Most types	1.5	160	13	18
Cocktails				
Bloody Mary	5	116	14	5
Daiquiri	2	111	14	2
Manhattan	2	178	17	2
Martini	2.5	156	22	trace
Old Fashioned	4	180	26	trace
Tom Collins	7.5	120	16	3

Source: Adapted from *Learning to Live Well with Diabetes* edited by Donnell D. Etzwiler, et al. (Diabetes Center, 1987).

to make, while the other was given the same basic instruction but not supervised as closely. After 4 years the two groups were compared and yes, the harder-working group had clearly reaped greater rewards. While 57 people in the more lax group had gone on to develop diabetes, only 26 in the more diligent group had—a significant difference indeed, the researchers said.

"This should be very encouraging news for people at high risk for developing type 2 diabetes, such as those with diabetes in the family or who have high blood pressure or are overweight," remarked the study's director, Jaakko Tuomilehto, M.D., a professor at the National Health Institute in Helsinki in response to the results.

ANSWERS TO FOOD QUESTIONS PEOPLE WITH DIABETES ASK MOST

"It's funny," says Daniel, age 51, diagnosed with type 2 diabetes 3 years ago. "The more I learn about this disease, the more questions I seem to have about it."

Find yourself in the same place? Good, because that's what the learning process is all about—becoming educated enough to begin to get a feel for all that you don't know. We offer the answers to the following questions in hopes of quenching at least part of that thirst.

Q. Is sugar a no-no for people with diabetes or not?

A. In its latest dietary guidelines, the ADA answers that question this way: "Scientific evidence has shown that the use of sucrose [table sugar] as part of the total carbohydrate content of the diet does not impair glucose control in individuals with type 1 or type 2 diabetes." The ADA hastens to add, however, that "sucrose and other sucrose foods must be substituted for other carbohydrates gram for gram and not simply added to the meal plan." So yes, sugar is permissible, but its carbohydrates—even though they've been found to raise blood sugar no more than the carbohydrates in bread, rice, or potatoes—

still must be accounted for in the overall balance of your diet. Considering that sugar is void of any beneficial nutrients, moreover, you would be wiser to get your carbohydrates from other more nutritious sources such as fruits, vegetables, and whole grains.

> *The use of sucrose (table sugar) as part of the total carbohydrate content of the diet does not impair glucose control in individuals with type 1 or type 2 diabetes.*

Q. I'm still confused about all the different types of sugar substitutes. Which are best for people with diabetes, and why?

A. Sugar substitutes fall into several basic categories. There are those (including corn syrup, honey, molasses, dextrose, and maltose) that contain the same calories and carbohydrates as sugar (sucrose) and hence cause essentially the same blood sugar responses as sugar. Another category of sweeteners are those that contain about half as many calories and carbohydrates as sugar (including sorbitol, mannitol, and xylitol) and hence produce about half the blood sugar response. A third category comprises the "nonnutritive" sweeteners that have no appreciable calorie or carbohydrate content at all and hence produce no appreciable blood sugar effects, either. These include saccharin, aspartame, acesulfame K, and sucralose. In a fourth category by itself is fructose (the type of sugar prevalent in fruits and vegetables), which, despite having a caloric content equal to that of sugar, does not cause blood sugar to rise as rapidly.

So which sweeteners are best? For purposes of controlling blood sugar as well as caloric intake, the nonnutritive category would have to get the nod.

Q. Do people with diabetes need to avoid fat more so than most people?

A. Yes. Diets high in fat (and the saturated fat in meats and full-fat dairy products, especially) are unhealthful for everyone, but people with diabetes need to be especially vigilant against these fats for several reasons: Not only can high-fat foods contribute to weight gain—thus worsening insulin insensitivity as well as increasing risks of high blood pressure—diets high in fat also tend to increase levels of triglycerides and LDL cholesterol in the blood, thus increasing risks for heart attacks and strokes, which pose special risks for people with diabetes already. This doesn't mean avoiding fat entirely, but it does mean exercising moderation and trying to get your fats in seafood, nuts, and oils such as olive, canola, or corn, whose fats are of the monounsaturated or polyunsaturated rather than unhealthful saturated variety.

Q. Do people with diabetes need to be especially careful to limit their intake of sodium?

A. Not necessarily. If high blood pressure is present, then, yes, care should be taken to limit sodium intake to less than 2,000 milligrams a day. If high blood pressure is not a problem, however, people with diabetes should observe the same recommendation made for most Americans, which is to keep sodium intake to under 3,000 milligrams a day. (Canned soups, canned vegetables, smoked meats, processed cheeses, crackers, pretzels, and chips tend to be highest in sodium, which you'll learn as you begin reading nutritional labels to sniff out the greatest sodium villains.)

> *If high blood pressure is not a problem, people with diabetes should observe the same sodium recommendation made for most Americans: under 3,000 milligrams a day.*

Q. Are there vitamins or other nutritional supplements that can be helpful for people with diabetes?

A. We'll be examining this question in more detail in chapter 7, but for now we'll simply say that the ADA's official position is no, nutritional supplements shouldn't be necessary for people with diabetes as long as they're eating the well-balanced diet the ADA recommends.

Some recent studies have been suggesting, however, that additional intake of certain nutrients—especially the antioxidant vitamins C and E—may help prevent some long-term complications of diabetes such as cataracts, retinopathy, nerve disorders, and blood vessel problems that can lead to heart attacks and strokes. There also is some evidence that certain mineral deficiencies may develop in some people with diabetes—shortages of magnesium, potassium, and possibly chromium, for example—which some experts feel supplements may help correct. As always, be sure to check with your doctor before giving any nutritional aid a try.

Q. **Can any herbs be helpful in controlling diabetes?**

A. Again, check chapter 7 for the full scoop, but yes, some research is beginning to suggest that certain herbs may be helpful in controlling glucose levels, with garlic, St. John's wort, *Aloe vera*, *Echinacea*, *Ginkgo biloba*, ginseng, fenugreek, primrose oil, and bilberry being considered among the most promising.

Q. **Can extra fiber in the diet help control the high blood sugar levels of diabetes?**

A. As with nutritional supplements and herbs, discoveries in this area remain in a somewhat controversial stage. The official position of the ADA is that no, the normal 20 to 35 grams of fiber recommended daily for most Americans is enough, but new research indicates more may be better. In a study done recently at the University of Texas and reported in the *New England Journal of Medicine*, for example, patients exhibited lower blood sugar as well triglyceride and cholesterol levels after 6 weeks of a diet that was twice as high in fiber as the ADA's recommendation. Soluble fiber—the gel-like type most prevalent in fruits, vegetables, and beans—is the type suspected of being most responsible for these beneficial effects.

START YOUR GLUCOSE CONTROL AT THE SUPERMARKET

It might seem obvious that we can't eat what we haven't bought, but our growing rates of obesity in America today would suggest that it's not been obvious enough. We need to learn to shop with our heads, not our salivary glands, nutritionists say, and we've got to stop being so easily swayed by food advertising, too. Easier said than done? Not if you employ these strategies—ways to shop as wisely as you know you should no matter what your stomach might have to say:

- **Have a plan—and stick to it.** This means no spur-of-the-moment deviations no matter how great the bargain: Cupcakes on sale are still cupcakes. Make up your shopping list when you're in your most rational mood of the day, and honor it no matter what.

- **If you shop with children, let them know who's boss.** Besides, it's a good idea for children to learn about good nutrition as early as possible, so tell your children *why* you're buying the foods you are—and maybe quiz them on subsequent visits to be sure it's sinking in.

- **Do not shop when you're hungry.** Hunger can gobble up even the best of intentions, so try to eat before you shop rather than after. You might even want to check your blood sugar before you head out to be sure it's going to be able to remain high enough to endure your trip. Should it fall low, your resulting hunger could encourage you to make unwise decisions—as could the impaired judgment low blood sugar can cause.

- **Head temptation off at the pass.** This means avoiding those aisles offering items with the greatest potential for testing your resolve. No shortcuts through the cookie aisle, even if it is the fastest way to the produce. The extra walk, moreover, will do you good.

Be a Fan of Fiber

If nutrients could run for office, fiber would be president. The list of medical conditions fiber has been alleged to remedy reads like a who's who of what ails us: obesity, heart disease, breast and colon cancer, constipation, hemorrhoids, diverticulosis, varicose veins, irritable bowel syndrome, gallstones—and yes, diabetes. They all can be helped to some degree by foods high in fiber. With respect to diabetes, foods high in fiber can help treat the disease as well as aid in preventing its onset.

In two large-scale population studies done by researchers from Harvard, for example, it was found that as people's consumption of high-fiber foods went up, their risks for developing type 2 diabetes tended to go down. And in research involving people already diagnosed with diabetes, James W. Anderson, M.D., of the University of Kentucky College of Medicine, found that a high-fiber diet helped people with type 2 diabetes improve their blood sugar control by 95 percent. People with type 1 diabetes were helped by 30 percent—not bad for a nutrient that doesn't even get digested.

But then that's how fiber works. In both of its two basic forms—soluble and insoluble—fiber is unique in that much of the good it

- **Be wary of foods marked "dietetic," "diabetic," or "sugar-free."** These foods may contain other sweetening agents that can make them just as loaded with calories and carbohydrates as their normal counterparts. Always check a food's nutritional label to be sure of exactly what you're getting.

- **Know the best of the basics.** Even shopping for such staples as bread, milk, and cereal can require some know-how to make the best choices possible. For example:

does comes from its ability to exit the body in basically the same chemical condition as it entered.

Soluble fiber—the kind found largely in fruits, vegetables, beans, and oatmeal—works to control blood glucose as well as blood cholesterol by creating a gel-like substance that coats the intestines and their contents, thus inhibiting the absorption of these two potential troublemakers into the bloodstream.

Insoluble fiber—the kind found mostly in wheat bran, whole grain cereals and breads, and the skins of fruits and vegetables—works its good deeds primarily by providing the dietary bulk needed not just to provide feelings of fullness, but also to move foods speedily through the intestines, thus reducing risks of constipation as well as hastening the exit of potential carcinogens that otherwise might linger in the intestinal tract.

Do you need to worry about making separate efforts to include more of these two types of fiber in your diet? Not really. Most foods high in fiber contain goodly amounts of both types, so by including lots of fresh fruits, vegetables, whole grain foods, beans, nuts, and seeds in your diet, you'll be covering both your soluble and insoluble fiber bases.

Bread. Choose varieties that list a whole grain flour as their first ingredient and offer at least 2 grams of fiber per serving.

Milk. Opt for 1 percent fat or skim.

Cereals. Go for brands that offer at least 3 grams of fiber, less than 5 grams of sugar, and less than 1 gram of fat per serving. (Oatmeal and most high-fiber cereals fit the bill.)

Rice. Highest in fiber are the wild, brown, and converted varieties. Basmati rice, research has shown, is an especially good choice for blood sugar control.

Cheese. Try to develop a taste for low- or non-fat varieties with 6 grams of fat or less per serving.

Beef. The higher the price, generally, the higher the fat, so choose cuts marked "select" or "choice" rather than "prime."

Poultry. Buy skinless, or remove the skin before cooking. You can reduce the fat content of most poultry products by 50 to 75 percent by doing so.

Luncheon meats. Unless they're marked at least 95 percent fat-free, keep shopping.

Canned fish. Opt for varieties packed in water rather than oil.

Vegetables. Go for fresh or frozen over canned.

Fruits and fruit juice. Again, choose fresh or frozen over canned, and make sure juices are marked "made with 100 per-cent pure juice."

Cookies and cakes. Spend a little time and you should be able to find varieties with less than 3 grams of fat per 100 calorie serving and still a lot of great taste.

Salad dressings. There's no shortage of great tasting low- and non-fat options.

THE LEGAL SPLURGE: MASTERING THE "EARNING" CURVE

No eating plan is going to be acceptable or even healthful if it leaves you with visions of sugar plums, not to mention devil's food cake dancing through your head. Nutritionists have come to realize this, and are now working with patients to help them learn the fine art of "just saying yes" when such cravings arise. The key lies in learning to *earn* your indulgences. By cutting back on your carbohydrate and fat intake at other times during the day to compensate, and perhaps adding some extra exercise to your normal routine, you should be able to have your splurges without consequence—or guilt, either.

Talk to your doctor about what this "earning" process might involve in your particular case, and especially if you take insulin or other medication that may need to be adjusted to make allowance for your regalement. Also be sure to test your blood sugar to be certain your levels are, in fact, under control after a special treat. If you play your cards right, however, you should be problem-free. "There really isn't any food that in moderation should have to be off-limits for anyone with diabetes," says Marion J. Franz, M.S., a registered dietician with the International Diabetes Center in Minneapolis.

> *B*y cutting back on your carbohydrate and fat intake at other times during the day to compensate, you should be able to have your splurges.

Ben and Jerry, Dolly Madison, and Sara Lee certainly should be happy to hear about that.

CHAPTER 6

The Elixir
Called Exercise

⤳

Thorough the idea of using exercise to treat diabetes is not new. Healers in China recommended exercise as a remedy for diabetes 1,500 years ago, and in this chapter we'll discover why. We'll see how exercise can help control diabetes by getting to the heart of what causes the disease in the first place—the body's inability to use glucose for energy. "Think of an exercising muscle as being like a glucose sponge," says Warren A. Scott, M.D., the medical director of Sportsmedicine of Soquel in California. "Vigorous exercise can cause muscles to increase their glucose uptake by as much as twentyfold, acting much like insulin in getting muscle cells to open up their glucose doors."

And the all-important end result of this boost in glucose uptake, of course, is less glucose in the blood—and hence fewer risks of the health problems excess glucose can cause. Exercise can be so effective in its insulin-like action, in fact, that it can help many people with type 2 diabetes eliminate their needs for medication entirely, while for those with type 1 diabetes it can reduce their insulin needs by as much as 50 percent.

But exercise can do more than just help control blood sugar; it can help lower triglycerides, blood pressure, and "bad" LDL cholesterol (while raising "good" HDL cholesterol), thus reducing the increased risks people with diabetes face for heart attacks and strokes. And as a calorie burner, and for some people an appetite suppressant, exercise can be just what the doctor ordered for the all-important goal of controlling weight. Regular exercise can even reduce risks of such major health problems as osteoporosis, arthritis, low back pain, and certain forms of cancer while also bolstering the immune system. It's definitely got the entire human body in mind when handing out its multiple gifts.

Think of an exercising muscle as being like a glucose sponge. Vigorous exercise can cause muscles to increase their glucose uptake by as much as twentyfold.

Nor does exercise forget the brain with its rewards, Dr. Scott points out, helping combat anxiety, depression, and emotional stress while building self-esteem. "Exercise gives people a sense of empowerment over their disease," Dr. Scott says. "It shows them they can do something very tangible about their condition, and something that makes them look better and feel better, too. In all the years I've worked with this disease, I'm still amazed at how much better patients do when they make regular exercise an important part of their lives, mentally as well as physically. It seems to give them added interest and energy in every other aspect of their treatment."

So let's take a look at exactly how exercise goes about working its metabolic as well as mental "miracles." It's high drama on a cellular level, as we'll see. Then we'll examine the easiest, safest, and most effective ways to fit exercise into your life. Yes, exercise requires more effort than just taking a pill, but the good news is that new research has found that this effort needn't be as strenuous or time consuming as previously thought. If there's new hope in the area of exercise, in fact, this is it: Scientists have found that the "medicine" called exercise doesn't have to be so hard to take after all. The old credo of "no pain, no gain" has been shown to be all wet in its own sweat. Controlling your diabetes with exercise can be as pain-free as a walk in the park or a bike ride with the kids. It's the consistency of your exercise efforts that counts, more so than the intensity, the new research shows. And as we'll see, those efforts can count a lot.

EXERCISE UNDER THE MICROSCOPE

So what really goes on inside the body of someone with diabetes who exercises regularly?

Boot up your imagination, allow some poetic license, and picture the following scenario. Envision a molecule of glucose drifting along in the bloodstream of someone with type 2 diabetes when it happens to encounter a muscle cell helping the person take a 3-mile walk. Normally the glucose molecule might have reason to be wary of getting too close to the muscle cell, because in a healthy body muscle cells consume glucose for energy. But the word has gotten out that the host of this muscle cell has diabetes, so the glucose molecule feels no fear.

It's the consistency of your exercise efforts that counts, more so than the intensity.

"Trying to get in shape there, chubbo?" the glucose teases.

"Yeah, but it's just a leisurely walk," the muscle cell replies, trying not to smirk. "I've been out of shape for quite a while, you know, so I don't want to overdo it."

Feeling even bolder, the glucose molecule moves closer to continue its taunt. "You diabetic cells are such wimps," it chides. "You've got no energy, no appetites, and you cause your host so many problems that you really ought to . . ."

"Ought to what?" the muscle cell asks as it suddenly opens its glucose portals and watches the glucose molecule begin to get sucked toward its demise. "Care to join me for lunch?"

Which the glucose molecule does—against its will, of course—permitting the muscle cell a small burp and a smile. "A little mustard would have been nice, but not bad. Maybe I'll go 4 miles now."

The moral of the story? Don't underestimate the power of exercise to give diabetic cells back their glucose appetites. As mentioned, exercise can increase the glucose uptake of muscle cells by as much as twentyfold, so it can be potent medicine indeed. Many experts, in fact, feel that in conjunction with proper diet, regular exercise could help 90 percent of people with type 2 diabetes discontinue medication entirely, while also helping them to normalize their blood pressure and blood fats. "In terms of a cure for type 2 diabetes, you might say exercise comes about as close right now as anything else we've got," says Dr. Scott.

> *I*n conjunction with proper diet, regular exercise could help 90 percent of people with type 2 diabetes discontinue medication entirely.

REGULAR MORE IMPORTANT THAN RIGOROUS

The closer scientists look at the benefits of exercise, in fact, the more they like what they see. "The benefits of regular exercise might sound almost too good to be true, but this is one miracle cure that really lives up to its advertising," write the editors of the *American Diabetes Association Complete Guide to Diabetes*.

Note, however, the word *regular* in the ADA's praise. With exercise, as with diet, consistency is the key. Studies show that the improvements in insulin sensitivity that result from an exercise session are capable of lasting perhaps 2 days at best. After that, like Cinderella at midnight, insulin sensitivity reverts back to preexercise levels. Other longer-term benefits of exercise, such as greater physical endurance, improved flexibility, lower blood fats, and increased muscle mass, endure beyond this 2-day window, of course, but even these gains are attained faster and maintained better when exercise is done on a regular as opposed to "when it fits" basis.

This is something to remember as you contemplate what might be the best exercise program for you. If it's not something you're going to be able to do at least three to five times a week—*every week*—you'd better return to the drawing board. Research shows that exercising daily is best of all for managing diabetes, in fact, so with this in mind you should put high priorities on convenience, practicality, and *fun*. Do not make the mistake of choosing an exercise routine you're only going to abandon out of inconvenience or boredom. By being active in ways you enjoy, you'll be active more often, and your exercise will do you a lot more good. *The consistency of your efforts, remember, is more important than their intensity.*

> *B*y being active in ways you enjoy, you'll be active more often, and your exercise will do you a lot more good.

Remember, too, that one of the greatest benefits of exercise in combating diabetes is its potential for elevating mood and stress—yet another reason to exercise in ways you enjoy. "The stress just of having diabetes can be plenty without patients having to worry about workouts they dread," Dr. Scott says. "I try to help my patients come up with the most enjoyable and useful exercise routines they can, so that exercise can help relieve their stress rather than add to it. A walk on Monday, cutting the grass on Tuesday, maybe a game of tennis on Wednesday—that kind of thing. As long as people are up and moving, they're doing so much more good for themselves than just sitting around.

"The fitness concepts of the 1970s and 1980s created an all-or-nothing attitude that I think some of us still are having trouble getting over today," Dr. Scott adds. "We think that if we haven't broken a major sweat we haven't done any good, but that's just not true."

LESS PAIN, MORE GAIN

If all this is beginning to sound like a green light to "do your own thing" to get the exercise you need, it is. And the permission is coming not just from Dr. Scott but from the top health organizations in the country—including the National Institutes for Health, the

The Anatomy of a Workout

Not the exercise type? You might want to think about turning over a new leaf—or at least raking a few. Studies show that even by including more moderate-intensity activities in your life, such as yard work or household chores, you confront head-on the very metabolic problems responsible for type 2 diabetes in the first place. Regular exercise can aid glucose control—while also reducing risks of heart attacks and strokes—in the following ways:

- **Exercise makes the body more sensitive to injected insulin, and also its own.** Exercise does this by increasing not just the sensitivity of existing insulin receptor sites on the body's muscle cells but also by creating new ones. For people with type 1 diabetes, this can mean substantial reductions in insulin needs, and for as many as 90 percent of people with type 2 diabetes, it could help them eliminate their medication needs entirely.

- **Exercise makes the body better at storing glucose in the muscles and liver.** This is important because more glucose stored in the liver and muscles means less glucose in the blood and hence less risk for the myriad of complications excess blood glucose can cause.

- **Exercise can help rid the body of excess fat.** This is critical for several reasons. Not only does losing body fat help restore

Centers for Disease Control and Prevention, the Office of the Surgeon General, the American Council on Exercise, and the American College of Sports Medicine. Any exercise program you're considering will need to be discussed with your doctor, of course, and the more closely the program can be tailored to meet your particular condition and needs, the safer and more effective it will be. But some general exercise recommendations have been emerging from these

insulin sensitivity; it can help lower blood pressure and blood fats—both primary risk factors for the cardiovascular complications diabetes can pose if left uncontrolled.

- **Exercise can help increase muscle mass.** More muscle mass means glucose in the blood must face more "hungry mouths" to feed. This is especially helpful for many people with type 2 diabetes because in addition to reducing the tissue damage that high glucose levels can cause, less glucose means the pancreas will need to produce less insulin, thus reducing risks for high blood pressure, high blood fats, and weight gain that can result from too much of this fat-storing hormone. More muscle mass also means a higher metabolic rate and hence greater calorie-burning even when your body is at rest.

- **Exercise can combat depression and elevate self-esteem.** Many experts feel that this may be the greatest benefit of all because without a winning attitude, all other aspects of treatment become that much more difficult to pursue. Exercise can elevate mood by helping the body release its own feel-good chemicals called *endorphins*. It also does so by giving us proof—whether in the form of lower blood fats or a thinner waist—that what we're doing is actually having some measurable effects.

leading health organizations recently that are important for you and your health care team to consider—important because they reflect significant changes in what healthful exercise is thought to require. The exercise "pill," you might say, has been made easier to swallow.

Out the window, for example, go what have been the two greatest stumbling blocks to greater exercise participation by Americans today. Our current activity levels are as low as they are (only about 20 percent of us get the exercise we need to cover all our health bases, surveys show) because we find exercise too time-consuming and too boring—excuses we're now going to find a lot harder to use. According to the new exercise guidelines, we may use practically any "moderate-intensity" activity we want for exercise just as long as we burn an extra 150 calories a day doing it. Better yet, we may pursue these activities in bits and pieces—individual sessions as short as just 10 minutes each, in fact—rather than worrying about exercising vigorously for 30 minutes at a stretch.

> *We may pursue exercise in bits and pieces—individual sessions as short as just 10 minutes each—rather than worrying about exercising vigorously for at least 30 minutes at a stretch.*

What these new guidelines mean is that we can now enjoy the "gains" of exercise without the "pain" of having to set aside huge blocks of time or even of having to break a sweat. Officials from the National Institutes of Health report that most of us still have a long way to go to get the amount of exercise we need to cover even our most basic health needs, but these new guidelines should go a long way to shrink that number, and some waistlines, as well. Most experts now agree that the former exercise guidelines that required our exercise sessions to last at least 20 to 30 minutes did more to alienate would-be exercisers than to include them—a situation these experts now hope the new guidelines will help correct. As admitted by the panel of experts assembled by the NIH, "Current low rates of regular activity in Americans may be partially due to the misperception that vigorous, continuous exercise is necessary to reap health benefits."

So banish such thoughts. Forget "no pain, no gain" and try this new fitness credo on for size instead: "Let fun get it done!" That's right. Scientists are now allowing us a kinder and gentler way. The latest studies show that simply by putting together approximately 30 minutes a day of activities as pleasurable and practical as walking the dog, washing the car, or beating a friend in a game of badminton, we can reduce our risks of virtually every major health problem we face today—the complications of diabetes included.

> ### Have a Minute to Live Longer?
> The next time you see a set of stairs, for example, don't pass them by for the escalator or elevator. In a study done at the University of Ulster in Ireland, college-aged women who fit 13 minutes of climbing stairs into their day for 7 weeks improved their fitness and upped their healthful HDL cholesterol levels by margins sufficient to reduce risks of heart disease by 33 percent. Two doctors from Johns Hopkins University reporting in the *New England Journal of Medicine,* moreover, have calculated that most of us could earn as much as an extra 4 seconds of life for every *single step* we climb!

THE HAZARDS OF NONE

The discussion thus far shouldn't imply that exercising more strenuously or for longer periods is bad, because it's not. It can be very good, in fact, for both people who have diabetes and those who don't. Richard K. Bernstein, M.D., for example, the author of *Dr. Bernstein's Diabetes Solution* and someone who's had type 1 diabetes for more than 50 years, has managed to keep himself incredibly robust in his late 60s with workouts based on strength training that he admits are quite strenuous. If you're a person who likes to sweat and would relish such a challenge, by all means talk to your doctor or an exercise physiologist about the possibilities that rigorous exercise has to offer. After all, Gary Hall Jr., who has type 1 diabetes, turned his diabetes into Olympic gold (see sidebar, "Diabetes Finds Gold in Swimmer Gary Hall," pages 180 and 181).

For most people with diabetes, however, just going from being sedentary to modestly active is where the greatest challenge lies and where the greatest benefits stand to be gained. Many large-scale studies show that the people who stand to gain most from exercise, in fact, are the one's who've been exercising the least, so anyone wanting to use this for motivation certainly is welcome to do so. To be avoided at all cost, the new research shows, is getting no exercise at all, which currently includes approximately 20 percent of Americans, and which poses the

Diabetes Finds Gold in Swimmer Gary Hall

To most people, being told you have type 1 diabetes as you're preparing for the greatest athletic challenge of your life would not seem conducive to a winning attitude. But then swimmer Gary Hall is not most people, so he won anyway—two gold medals plus a silver and a bronze at the 2000 Olympic Games in Sydney, just 18 months after being diagnosed. "The doctor who did my tests told me my swimming career was over," the 26-year-old Hall now recalls in the *Sports Illustrated* online article, "A Chance to Encourage Millions."

Two more doctors also told Gary his career was sunk, but Gary kept shopping, finally making contact with a physician who would buoy his hopes and assist him in his quest. She was Anne Peters, M.D., now the director of clinical diabetes at the University of Southern California Keck School of Medicine, and they clicked. Dr. Peters understood his frustration and his passion, so they set out to prove the medical world wrong. "I wanted to show people this is something you can cope with," Hall says.

At first the coping didn't come easily. For 2 months following his diagnosis and before finding Dr. Peters, Gary went through a deep depression, feeling angry, scared, and confused. "My first reaction when I was diagnosed was a desire to fall down, and I wasn't even standing," Gary recalls. "I couldn't believe it. I thought that diabetes was a disease that happened only to old people who had neglected their health for more years than I had even been alive. I was upset in

same risks for early death as—are you ready for this?—smoking a pack of cigarettes a day.

Yikes is right. It seems the butts we sit on may be as hazardous to our health as the ones we smoke. Lack of physical activity has been estimated to play a role in as many as 250,000 premature deaths in

every sense of the word. Dumfounded, horrified, furious, and depressed, but most of all, really scared."

"Why me?" was the big question Gary kept asking himself, but as he learned more about his disease, he began to arrive at an answer. He had a chance to show the world that diabetes didn't have to be a dream wrecker, even when those dreams were of Olympic gold. So he got back in the pool, and with Dr. Peters coaching his every move, did some of the best training in his life. He also put his heart and soul into his treatment, monitoring his blood sugar as often as 10 times a day to be assured of being at his metabolic best. "It got to where I could just squeeze my fingers and get blood," he says of the pincushions his digits had become.

But the hard work paid off—and quickly. Within just 5 months of being diagnosed, Gary swam the fastest 50 meters of his life, good enough for first place at the national championships and a new American record.

"That's when it really hit me," Gary says. "I realized I had a chance to encourage millions of people living and suffering with this disease, a chance to help people of all ages conquer their feelings of helplessness and defeat. I figured if I was able to do that, even just for one person, it would be an accomplishment far greater than anything I'd ever be able to achieve in the pool."

Gary's athletic accomplishment is now Olympic history—two gold medals plus a silver and a bronze—but the success of his other goal remains to be determined by people like you.

the United States each year, in fact—about 12 percent of the total—so being a "couch potato" really isn't something to joke about. We live in bodies that were born to move, and we do them a great disservice when we don't allow them to do so. As the list in the "Good for More Than Just Diabetes" sidebar shows, exercise is not just for getting "buffed"; it's for keeping the body's most basic systems operating as they should. Many experts feel that lack of exercise may be an underappreciated factor in many of our most chronic and serious health problems today.

> *Getting no exercise at all poses the same risks for early death as smoking a pack of cigarettes a day.*

BUT CAN "NICE AND EASY" DO IT FOR DIABETES, TOO?

This question, first of all, is best answered by your doctor with respect to your particular condition because no two cases of diabetes are alike. Given the circumstances of most type 2 cases, however, the new, more permissive guidelines allow for the very sort of flexibility that most experts feel patients need in order to make exercise a regular part of their lives.

"As long as people keep good track of their blood sugars and eat appropriately to accommodate their exercise, these new guidelines are great because they allow patients to get the exercise they need in ways that work best for them," says Guy Hornsby, Ph.D., a certified diabetes educator and associate chair of exercise physiology at West Virginia University.

Other experts agree. Robert Hanisch, for example, a certified diabetes educator and certified strength and conditioning specialist at the Diabetes Treatment Center at Columbia Hospital in Milwaukee, has been testing the effects of short, moderate-intensity activity sessions on hundreds of patients with diabetes and has come up with highly encouraging results. "My research has shown that for most patients, even when exercise sessions are short, blood sugar levels

---

Good for More than Just Diabetes

Pat yourself on the back for helping control more than just your diabetes when you become more active. You may pride yourself in reducing your risks for these common health problems as well:

Arthritis	Insomnia
Cancer (of the colon, prostate, female reproductive organs and breast)	Low back pain
	Menopause symptoms
	Obesity
	Osteoporosis
Constipation	Sexual dysfunction
Depression	Stress
Heart attacks and strokes	Susceptibility to illness and infection
High blood pressure	

---

will drop an average of about 1 to 2 points for every minute they spend exercising," he says. "This will vary, of course, depending on when they've last eaten or taken medication, but that's the average I've observed."

Blood sugar monitoring may become a little more complicated with this "bits and pieces" approach to exercise, Mr. Hanisch concedes, but patients shouldn't let this become an obstacle, especially if the only other option is to do no exercise at all. "What patients need to realize is that as long as several short sessions of activity expend the same amount of energy as a continuous longer session, the same overall reductions in glucose should occur," he says.

FORGET THE SWEAT

Any time you've got a few spare minutes, you've got an opportunity for a "workout," even if it's just mowing some grass or hanging up a load of wash. "Besides," Mr. Hanisch adds, "many people with type 2 diabetes have never exercised before in their lives, so any amount of exercise they get is going to be beneficial, and this is the message we need to get across. People need to stop approaching exercise with an all-or-nothing attitude because in truth, even a little is so much better than none at all."

What the new more permissive exercise guidelines do most of all, these experts agree, is to give patients more options. Under the old guidelines, if you didn't have at least a half hour or so to workout—not to mention time to take a shower—you didn't do anything at all. But now with the possibility of shorter and less strenuous exercise sessions, your options are limited only by your imagination. You can take a short walk, do some housework, or putter around the yard— with no need for a shower because you probably won't even be breaking a sweat!

> *For most patients, even when exercise sessions are short, blood sugar levels will drop an average of about 1 to 2 points for every minute.*

Better yet, the calories you burn at such miniworkouts will count every bit as much for weight control as those burned during longer exercise sessions, as the studies described in the next section show.

Minimal Workouts, Maximal Results: Short Can Be Sweet

Don't have time for one of those "30-minutes-or-don't-bother" exercise sessions of old? No problem. The following studies show that exercise programs composed of sessions as short as 10 minutes each can provide equal benefits, aiding weight loss, and contributing to a healthier heart:

- In a study lasting 8 weeks, done at the Stanford University School of Medicine, researchers found that middle-aged men who exercised three times a day for 10 minutes per session experienced essentially the same increases in maximum oxygen uptake (a measure of cardiovascular fitness) as men who exercised for 30 minutes continuously. "Multiple short bouts of moderate-intensity exercise training significantly increase peak oxygen uptake," concluded the researchers in their *American Journal of Cardiology* report.

- In a 20-week study of obese sedentary women done at the University of Pittsburgh Medical Center, scientists found that women who worked out on exercise equipment for 20 to 40 minutes daily by dividing their workouts into 10-minute segments were more successful at losing weight and sticking with their exercise programs than women who worked continuously for the same 20- to 40-minute period. "This study indicates that even 10-minute exercise sessions can be effective for weight control and are a good beginning for a lasting commitment to a healthy lifestyle," concluded the researchers at the Annual Meeting of the Society of Behavioral Medicine in 1998.

- Compared to women who walked for 30 minutes per session, women in a University of Nebraska study who walked twice a day for 15 minutes not only were twice as likely to stick with their programs but also wound up covering twice the mileage.

Because the body's metabolism remains accelerated for a short time after an exercise session has ended, some research suggests this may give a weight loss advantage to working out several times rather than just once a day. "Think of exercise as being like spinning a wheel," says Robert Hanisch. "Calories will continue to be burned during the time it takes the wheel to slow back down."

Don't forget to get approval from your doctor before taking on any new level of physical activity, however, no matter how modest, and especially if it's been a while since you've last been active. This is particularly true if you're over 35 or have had diabetes for 10 years or more. As explained elsewhere in this chapter, certain conditions can require exercise to be approached with special caution.

Table 5. More Than One Way to Burn a Calorie

Activity	Calories Burned in 30 Minutes (for someone weighing 180 pounds)
Fun Activities	
Badminton	235
Dancing (ballroom)	145
Dancing (disco)	230
Golf (no cart)	205
Hiking (hilly terrain)	325
Horseback riding (trot)	250
Horseshoes	110
Racquetball	370
Scuba diving	340
Sex (moderately passionate)	120
Skating (inline or ice)	230
Skiing (cross-country)	335
Skiing (downhill)	230
Snowshoeing	405
Soccer	330
Squash	385
Table tennis (Ping-Pong)	170
Tennis (singles)	260
Tennis (doubles)	165
Volleyball	200

(continues)

Let Fun Get It Done

Does even just the thought of exercise make your heart beat faster? Relax. Exercise doesn't have to happen in a costly sweat suit or even make you sweat. The latest research shows you can cover your fitness bases simply by amassing 150 calories' (about 30 minutes) worth of moderate-intensity activity on most or all days of the week—no "pain" required. And don't worry if you can't burn those 150 calories

Walking (moderate pace)	150
Walking (brisk pace)	215
Water skiing	270
Practical Activities	
Gardening (digging and hoeing)	290
Gardening (weeding)	180
Mopping floors	150
Mowing grass (pushing a power mower)	245
Painting	190
Raking leaves	250
Scrubbing floors	260
Shoveling (light) snow	350
Stacking firewood	225
Trimming hedges (manual clippers)	190
Vacuuming	120
Washing windows	145
Washing/polishing car	140
Conventional Fitness Activities	
Cycling (moderate pace)	245
Jogging	378
Jumping rope	342
Rowing	280
Swimming (slow crawl)	315
Weight training	170

Source: Adapted from *Fitness Without Exercise* by Bryant Stamford, Ph.D., and Porter Shimer (Warner Books, 1990).

all at once. Studies show that activity sessions as short as 10 minutes can provide the same benefits as longer sessions as long as a daily total of 150 calories is burned.

Table 5 shows the approximate number of calories used for each of the activities listed. The numbers in this table are based on a person weighing 180 pounds. People who weigh more than 180 pounds will use slightly more calories in the same activity, while lighter people will use slightly fewer.

METABOLISMS OUT OF SHAPE

Exercise can be so helpful in treating type 2 diabetes, in fact, that many experts speculate that diabetes may be due in part to the general lack of exercise in today's high-tech world. "Type 2 diabetes is less common in physically active compared to inactive societies," notes professor of health and exercise science at Appalachian State University, David C. Nieman, Dr.PH. Studies also show that cultures formerly accustomed to active lifestyles, such as Native Americans, fall prey to diabetes at an alarming rate when they adopt the sedentary ways of the modern world.

Why should inactivity pose such significant risks? Because it doesn't allow us to use our bodies as they were designed, says Dr. Scott. "Think about it. Here we are with essentially the same biological makeup we had 50,000 years ago when we had to be active all day every day just to survive, and what do we do with them now? We sit. We sit while commuting to and from our jobs, we sit at our jobs, and we sit when we get home. The result, in a sense, is that the glucose in our bloodstreams has forgotten what it's supposed to do." So it accumulates and gets into trouble instead, gumming up the bloodstream and fouling nearly every biological system it encounters.

*W*e're putting more glucose into our bloodstreams than our out-of-tune engines can handle—and stalling out as a result.

This admittedly is a simplification of the intricate interplay between glucose and insulin that diabetes involves, Dr. Scott concedes, but the basic logic behind it is sound. "To use an automotive analogy, we're flooding our engines," Dr. Scott says. "We're putting more glucose into our bloodstreams than our out-of-tune engines can handle—and stalling out as a result."

It's a persuasive metaphor, especially since this "obsolescence" of physical activity in today's hyperautomated world has been so sudden and severe, giving our bodies little time to adapt. As recently as a hundred years ago, for example, fully one-third of the energy responsible for powering the U.S. economy came from human muscle—a figure that now is down to less than 1 percent. Given the parade of energy-sparing gadgets ranging from electric-knives to dust busters that also have been encroaching on our energy expenditures at home, it's no wonder diabetes has been on such a rampage. Our muscles, you might say, have suffered the greatest "layoff" of all.

Nor has the fitness "boom" succeeded in rectifying our dilemma, despite what all the athletic shoe and sports beverage commercials would have us believe. Obesity is a considerably larger problem today, in fact, than before all the huffing and puffing in the name of health was kicked off by Dr. Ken Cooper's runaway bestseller *Aerobics* back in 1968. "When substance is separated from hype, the fitness boom was a national obsession that for most of us never translated into a way of life," *Walking* magazine has commented on the fitness boom's fizzle.

The boom, you might say, was a "bust," so don't feel bad if it passed you by. You can catch up, starting now, simply by putting together 30 minutes of moderate-intensity activities a day.

EXERCISE FOR THE OBESE

It's no secret that type 2 diabetes goes hand-in-hand with being overweight. By making the body less sensitive to insulin, excess body fat has much to with the development of type 2 diabetes in the first place, especially if the excess fat is carried largely in the area of the abdomen, research shows. Worse yet, being overweight in people with type 2 diabetes can begin to compound itself as insulin insensitivity that often causes the body to produce more insulin than it should in an attempt to compensate. This is unfortunate, given that insulin is the body's chief fat-storing hormone. Type 2 diabetes, therefore, could be said to be its own worst enemy by exacerbating the very conditions at the heart of its cause—a cycle that only weight loss, preferably aided by exercise, can break.

Exercise for Preventing Diabetes: Hard to Hit a Moving Target

For many of the same reasons exercise can help treat diabetes, it may be able to prevent it. The body's cells need to be kept sensitive to insulin, and the muscles and liver need to be kept in "shape" for storing glucose (as glycogen), thus helping keep excess glucose out of the blood. Body fat—and abdominal fat especially—also needs to be kept in check to keep cells responsive to insulin's effects.

Might exercise be just what the doctor ordered for all of the above? The results of the following studies would suggest it certainly can help:

- In a 14-year study of more than 6,000 male alumni of the University of Pennsylvania, Dr. Ralph Paffenbarger of Stanford University found that the risk for developing diabetes for men who were lean and active was only one-quarter as great as for men who were inactive and obese.

- In a study that charted the health of more than 87,000 nurses for eight years, Dr. JoAnn Manson of the Harvard Medical School and Brigham and Women's Hospital in Boston found that women who exercised at least once a week were 33 percent less likely to develop diabetes than women who were

But obesity in the person with type 2 diabetes offers yet another nasty "closed feedback loop," as this type of cycle is known in scientific terms. The heavier people get, the less amenable to exercise they generally become, thus further galvanizing their fate. Not only does exercise become progressively less comfortable from a physical standpoint, it tends to become less comfortable from a psychological standpoint, too, as increasing weight begins to erode self-esteem. The result is two vicious cycles working at once—a physical one and a psy-

inactive. Dr. Manson found similar results in her 5-year study of over 21,000 men: Those who were physically active were at a 36 percent reduced risk for diabetes than men who were not active.

- Researchers from Great Britain found after studying 7,735 men for 13 years that the most active, compared to the least active, had reduced their risks for developing diabetes by over 50 percent.

- In Finland, researchers found that men who exercised at least 40 minutes a week reduced their diabetes risks by 64 percent compared to men who did not exercise at all.

- In a 6-year study of nearly 7,000 men in Hawaii, those who were the most active were found to have less than half the risk for developing diabetes than the least active men even after adjustments were made for age, obesity, family history, and other factors known to influence diabetes onset.

So what's the bottom line? Diabetes has a lot more difficulty catching up to a "moving" target.

chological one—creating a veritable "figure eight" of negativity that has to be broken if progress against type 2 diabetes is to be made.

If this is striking any personal chords, perhaps the following advice can help. In combination with proper dietary measures, exercise is critical for creating the metabolic changes that can make the difference between success and failure in a weight-loss campaign. The tips come from Bryant Stamford, Ph.D., who has helped thousands of overweight people tip the scales in their favor over the years in his role as the director of the Health Promotion and Wellness Center at the University of Louisville in Kentucky.

> *The heavier that people get, the less amenable to exercise they generally become, thus further galvanizing their fate.*

- **Let your comfort be your guide.** Don't make the mistake of thinking that because you're overweight you have to work that much harder to catch up to the pack. You should take just the opposite approach, in fact, so that your first efforts won't leave you feeling discouraged or so sore you're ready to throw in the towel before even getting started. Whatever activity you choose, begin at a pace that leaves you sufficient wind to converse with someone comfortably, and stop to rest when you feel tired. Exercise does not have to be continuous to help you lose weight, remember, or to improve your health, either. It's the total number of calories you burn in a day that counts, not the amount of time it takes you to do it.

- **Enjoy your calorie-burning advantage.** Yes, laws of physics are on your side. The more weight you carry, the more calories you're going to burn at whatever you do. While someone weighing 130 pounds might burn 350 calories during an hour of mowing grass, for example, someone weighing 200 pounds would burn about 550, so let that put some wind in your weight-loss sails!

- **Keep cool.** People who are overweight need to be more careful to avoid becoming overheated when exercising because body fat is, in fact, a form of insulation. This can be done easily enough, however, by walking in air-conditioned malls during the summer, wearing light and loose-fitting clothing rather than sweat gear, and swimming or doing exercises in a pool if possible. Drinking plenty of water before, during, and after exercise also can help.

- **Take a load off**. Because extra pounds can put extra stress on weight-bearing joints such as the knees and ankles, some overweight exercisers find activities done from a sitting position such as cycling or rowing preferable to such mainstays as jogging, walking, and racquet sports.

- **Don't rely too heavily on willpower.** Some may be necessary, of course, but if you're having to rely too heavily on willpower, you might want to reexamine what you're doing for exercise. It should be something you enjoy enough so that major willpower isn't required.

- **Learn to bend so you won't break.** An all-or-nothing attitude can do more to crash a fitness program than many perfectionists realize. If you miss an exercise session or even several, tell yourself you're human and just get back on schedule when you can. It makes no sense whatsoever to punish yourself further by trashing your exercise program for good.

THE STRENGTHS OF STRENGTH TRAINING

Like aerobic exercise, the benefits of strength training also have become apparent (and not just for kicking sand in people's faces at the beach). Like aerobic exercise, strength training can help condition the heart and lungs and have positive effects on blood fats and blood pressure, but its greatest plus may be that it can help build muscle tissue and hence increase glucose uptake in addition to elevating calorie-burning 24 hours a day. Muscle demands more calories than fat, not just while it's active, you see, but also while it's at rest. The more muscle mass you have, therefore, the better you're going to be at burning calories—and controlling your weight—even as you're just watching the evening news.

Strength training can be especially valuable as we get older, moreover, because the aging process likes to take our muscle mass away, and our strength along with it. Studies show that the strength of the average American declines by about 20 percent between the ages of 30 and 65, and beyond the age of 65 the decline becomes an avalanche. After the age of 74, one-quarter of men and about two-thirds of women can't lift anything heavier than 10 pounds. So much for those piggyback rides for the grandkids or possibly any sizeable Christmas gifts, either.

> *Muscle demands more calories than fat, not just while it's active but also while it's at rest.*

Responsible for these declines is a wasting away of what are known as "fast-twitch" muscle fibers, and lack of use is the primary cause. The other type of muscle fibers we have—called "slow-twitch"—are called upon by activities as routine as walking and brushing our teeth, so just going about our normal day tends to keep these fibers reasonably well in tact. Not so with our fast-twitch fibers, however. Only activities that require considerable strength activate these, so unless we engage in such activities, our fast-twitch friends wither and eventually disappear altogether.

And that's you, you're afraid? Don't bet on it. Studies show that considerable gains in strength and muscle mass can be achieved by people who've been inactive most of their lives, even by folks in their 90s. In a study done at Tufts University, for example, men as old as 96 were able to triple their strength by weight training for a period of just 12 weeks. Subsequent studies, moreover, showed similar results were achievable by women.

Muscle cells are dying for a second chance, you might say, and it doesn't take being a dedicated body-builder to give it to them. Remember, too, that just as muscles burn more calories than fat, they also burn more glucose, so the more muscle you have, the easier it's going to be to keep your blood sugar—as well as those bullies at the beach—in check.

Even more so than aerobic exercise, in fact, strength training increases what are known as glucose transporters on the surface of the body's cells, thus facilitating glucose uptake, and these transporters develop not only on muscle cells but on other types of tissue as well. As a result, not just glucose control but also weight control becomes considerably easier for people who include muscle-building workouts in their exercise programs, says Richard K. Bernstein, M.D., in his book *Dr. Bernstein's Diabetes Solution*. "As you increase your muscle mass with strength training, you reduce your insulin needs," he explains, "and having less insulin in your bloodstream means you reduce the amount of fat your body stores."

> *As you increase your muscle mass with strength training, you reduce your insulin needs, and having less insulin in your bloodstream means you reduce the amount of fat your body stores.*
>
> —RICHARD K. BERNSTEIN, M.D.

Better Safe than Sorry

The benefits of strength training aren't without risks for certain people, however, so be sure to talk to your doctor before embarking on a program. Because the proper equipment can be quite expensive, moreover, and there are so many different exercises for different muscle groups that require proper technique and sequencing of repetitions and sets, it's best to get instruction at a gym or health club from a qualified instructor, Dr. Bernstein says.

Considering all of strength training's other benefits—such as helping preserve bone mass and providing protective strength to arthritis-prone joints—"pumping iron" can indeed be a worthwhile addition to your exercise program. Here are some basic guidelines from the ADA that can help keep this valuable form of exercise as safe as possible:

- **Check with your doctor before pumping as much as a single pound.** Certain diabetic complications such as nerve damage and eye and kidney problems can make strenuous exercise of any type inadvisable—strenuous strength-training, especially—so be sure to get an official go-ahead from your doctor.

- **Test your blood sugar before, during, and after strength training—just as you would with aerobic exercise—to avoid potentially dangerous blood sugar fluctuations.** You certainly wouldn't want to develop low blood sugar in the midst of a maximum bench press.

- **Do 5 to 10 minutes of light aerobic activity such as walking, slow jogging, or jumping rope as a warm-up.** Muscles that are warmed with an increased blood flow are less prone to strains.

- **Practice proper breathing by exhaling as you lift a weight and inhaling as you lower it.** Holding your breath during lifts may cause dangerous elevations in blood pressure.

- **Always do your weight-training with another person (a qualified trainer is best) to help out should an especially heavy weight catch you in a "pinch."** It happens more often than you may think, and especially to those looking for the greatest gains.

- **Allow at least 1 day of rest between strength workouts to allow for recuperation, or alternate workouts that exercise different muscle groups**—upper body muscles one day, for example, lower body the next. Don't waste those rest days, however—simply do something aerobic such as walking, cycling, or light yard or housework to keep your calorie burning on track and your insulin sensitivity in good tune.

WHAT ELSE EXERCISE IS GOOD FOR (ALL OF YOU)

When Aristotle observed back in 300 B.C., "We fall into ill health as a result of not caring to exercise," as usual, he knew what he was talking about. Exercise can be potent medicine for helping control the short-term high blood sugars of diabetes and for preventing many of its long-term complications as well. But exercise can do a lot more than just combat the potential ill effects of diabetes; it can be a health booster for all of you, as the following list shows:

- **Exercise is good for the blood.** In addition to reducing fat particles in the blood (triglycerides), regular exercise can boost healthful blood components called HDLs (high-density lipoproteins) that can reduce risks of heart attacks and strokes by helping keep fatty deposits from collection on artery walls. Regular exercise also can reduce the tendency of the blood to clot, which also can decrease stroke and heart attack risks.

- **Exercise is good for the blood vessels**. The blood vessels themselves also benefit from exercise as they become more elastic in response to the increased blood demands. Over time, even brand-new blood vessels can develop in response to this increased blood flow, thus helping oxygenate and nourish the body's cells even more.

- **Exercise is good for the joints**. Exercise can strengthen the muscles responsible for supporting and operating the body's joints, thus helping protect them from arthritis as well as injury.

- **Exercise is good for the bones.** Weight-bearing exercise such as walking, jogging, and weight-lifting strengthens the bones by creating electrical impulses that increase their uptake of calcium—important for avoiding osteoporosis.

- **Exercise is good for the muscles.** This might seem like a no-brainer, but it can be especially important as we age.

- **Exercise is good for the back.** Studies show that people who are regularly active have fewer back problems than people who are not—the result of greater strength in the muscles, including those of the abdomen, responsible for giving the spine its support.

- **Exercise is good for the skin.** By increasing supplies of oxygen and other vital nutrients to the skin by way of enhanced blood flow, exercise can make the skin more resistant to wrinkles by making it thicker and more elastic.

- **Exercise is good for weight control.** By increasing our ability to burn calories even while we're at rest—and also by helping keep our self-esteem in shape—exercise is more helpful for long-term weight control than any other tactic.

- **Exercise is good for the digestive system.** By helping the body absorb nutrients as well as promoting more regular bowel habits, exercise could be said to aid digestion from top to bottom.

- **Exercise is good for the immune system.** By stimulating the activity of T cells, moderate exercise may help protect against everything from colds and flu to skin infections and even certain cancers, some studies suggest.

- **Exercise is good for coordination and reaction time.** Not just athletes need these attributes; we all do for everything from safer driving to avoiding falls as we get up in our years.

- **Exercise is good for the sex drive.** Studies with men and women alike show that people who exercise have more active sex lives—and probably for physical and psychological reasons alike, researchers say.

- **Exercise is good for sleep.** People who are regularly active also report sleeping better—due probably to less physical tension and psychological stress, scientists say.

- **Exercise is good for the brain.** The same blood flow that's good for the body appears to be good for the brain as exercise has been associated with better cognitive function (including memory and problem solving), especially as we age.

- **Exercise is good for the spirits.** Whether by increasing production of our own feel-good brain chemicals called endorphins or by simply giving us a feeling of accomplishment, researchers aren't sure, but what is clear is that regular exercise has been shown to be a powerful antidote to depression, anxiety, and stress.

ARE YOU AN EXERCISE WASTER?

Because weight control is so important for managing type 2 diabetes, the more calories you can burn during the day, the better—regardless of how you do it. The more vigorous and prolonged an activity is, the more calories it will burn, of course, but this does not exclude the additive value of short spurts of moderate or even light-intensity activities that might not even impress you as worthy of the "exercise" label.

Are you letting such valuable exercise opportunities pass you by? Try your hand at this short quiz to find out. And if you do poorly, don't feel bad. You might consider it good news, in fact, because it means better fitness (and hence better blood sugar control) may be more available to you than you think. By capitalizing on more of these missed opportunities, in fact, you might burn as many as an extra 50 calories a day—enough for a loss of about 5 pounds in a year without having to add any "real" exercise to your life at all.

1. When watching TV, do you change channels using a remote rather than getting up and doing it the "old-fashioned" way?
   a) Yes, always.
   b) Usually, and especially when I'm feeling tired.
   c) I don't even own a TV remote.

2. When looking for a parking place, do you take whatever time is necessary to find the most convenient spot possible?
   a) Yes, always.
   b) Only if the weather is bad.
   c) No, because I realize the walking is good exercise.

3. When you're at home and want to say something to someone in another room, is it more your style to yell or to get up and speak to the person directly?

   a) I'm a yeller.

   b) It depends how far away the person is and how much I have to say.

   c) I think it's rude to yell, so I'll always make the effort to speak face-to-face.

4. When in an office building or department store, will you choose to take the stairs instead of an elevator or escalator?

   a) No, I hate to climb stairs because it leaves me breathless.

   b) If I have the time I will take the stairs.

   c) I never miss the opportunity to climb stairs because I know what super exercise it is.

5. Do you do your own house cleaning—or at least help—or do you hire this potential exercise away?

   a) I hire it away.

   b) I do as much as I have time to do.

   c) I do most or all of it and often break a pretty good sweat.

6. When doing something like taking out the garbage or unloading groceries from the car, will you burden yourself with an exceptionally clumsy load rather than make an extra trip?

   a) Yes, and it's not uncommon that I'll drop and break something.

   b) I will if I'm in a hurry or it's raining.

   c) No, I'll pretty much always make the extra trip.

7. Which word would you say best describes your collection of "power equipment"—indoor as well as outdoor, such as leaf blowers, hedge clippers, and handheld Dustbusters?

   a) State-of-the-art

   b) Average

   c) Skimpy

8. If you're having to wait for a long time at an airport, what will you do?
    a) Find the nearest snack bar or cocktail lounge.
    b) Read a magazine or book.
    c) Take a walk.

9. If you find yourself in an exceptionally long line at the check-out counter of a supermarket, what will you do?
    a) Start snacking on something in my cart.
    b) Check out one of the tabloids or make conversation.
    c) Do toe raises to work my leg muscles while I wait.

10. When you've finished unloading your groceries into your car, will you make an effort to return the cart to its central storage area outside the store?
    a) Heck no, that's what they pay those kids for.
    b) If I have time.
    c) Always.

Scoring

Give yourself 1 point for every *a* answer, 2 for every *b*, and 3 for each *c*.

24 to 30. Congratulations. You're not letting a moment of exercise escape you!

17 to 23. Not bad, but you could do better.

10 to 16. Shame on you. Your convenience could be inconveniencing your health.

MORE HEALTH, FEWER HAZARDS

Precisely because exercise can be such potent medicine, it needs to be used with a certain amount of know-how and caution to be as safe and beneficial as possible. Whether you plan to get your exercise by training for a marathon or just taking great care of your house or yard, therefore, you should follow some general guidelines.

As you might have guessed, it's very important to discuss any exercise you do with your doctor and maybe even an exercise specialist to be sure to get advice as specific to your particular condition as possible. "It's really best for each patient to be advised on a case-by-case basis with exercise," says Guy Hornsby, Ph.D., a diabetes educator and associate chair of exercise physiology at West Virginia University. "This is especially true for patients taking insulin, because dosages will need to be adjusted according to the intensity and duration of the exercise they do. Frequent glucose monitoring also is critical for getting the most from what exercise has to offer, and especially when just starting an exercise program to get the best idea possible of the effects it's having."

Exercise Guidelines

1. Get a thorough exam and your doctor's okay. This is especially important for people over 35 or who have had diabetes for more than 10 years. Some complications of diabetes such as eye disease, kidney disease, nerve damage, circulation problems, or heart disease may require special precautions or even make exercise inadvisable, so it's important to be examined thoroughly to be sure.

2. Consider consulting with a exercise physiologist who specializes in diabetes. Your doctor may even recommend it. An exercise specialist can be especially helpful with details such as appropriate exercise intensity and duration, blood sugar levels to look for before and after exercise, medication adjustments, injury prevention, and the best ways to accommodate your exercise through diet.

3. Begin slowly. This no doubt will be reinforced by your doctor and/or exercise consultant, but it can't hurt to make the point doubly clear here. It's important to give your body the time it needs to adapt to exercise, especially if you haven't been active for a while or are beginning an exercise program for the first time. Being active is something you want to make a lifetime habit, remember, so there's no sense in tripping yourself up at the very start. Better to be the tortoise than the hare.

4. Time exercise properly with meals. For most people with diabetes, the best time to exercise is about an hour after eating to assure that an adequate amount of glucose will be in the bloodstream to help fuel the activity. Waiting too long to exercise after eating—and hence without adequate glucose in the system—can run the risk of driving blood sugar levels too low, particularly if the activity is prolonged. Exercising too soon after eating, on the other hand, can cause indigestion or light-headedness as both the muscles of your body and the muscles of your stomach will be competing for the same blood supply.

5. Avoid exercising when medication is having its peak effects. This is true whether you're taking insulin, oral medications, or both, because the glucose-reducing effects of your medication in combination with the glucose-reducing effects of your exercise could get you into low-glucose trouble.

6. Test your glucose before, during, and after exercise. Testing this frequently is especially important in the beginning stages of an exercise program (or when trying a new activity for the first time) to help you determine how your body is responding. Tests done before exercise should be done about 30 minutes before the planned session and then again just before starting to determine whether blood sugar levels are rising, falling, or remaining fairly stable. If your levels are falling, you may need to fuel up with a small, low-fat, high-carbohydrate snack before exercising, such as a piece of fruit, some raisins, a few graham crackers, or 6 ounces or so of a nondiet soda. If blood sugar levels are high, on the other hand, insulin may be needed to bring levels to within a safe exercise range. Testing after exercise should be done as soon as possible after the session to get the truest reading of the effects the activity has had.

7. Avoid exercising when blood sugar levels are too high or too low. Exercising when blood sugar is too high (higher than about

250 milligrams/deciliter if ketones are present or about 300 milligrams/deciliter if they are not) can drive levels even higher because in the beginning stages, exercise can activate glucose stored in the muscles and liver. Exercising when blood sugar levels are too low, on the other hand, (less than about 100 milligrams/deciliter) can drive levels even lower as exercise gradually begins to draw on glucose supplies in the blood. These are general guidelines only, however, so be sure to check with your doctor to see what's best for you.

8. Know the healthiest postexercise glucose levels to shoot for. Again, check with your doctor on the best levels for your particular condition, but a healthy range is generally between 100 and 120 milligrams/deciliter for people taking insulin and between 80 and 120 milligrams/deciliter for people taking oral medication or no medication at all.

9. Don't exercise when you're sick. Not only can such overzealousness slow your recovery, but illness usually alters glucose levels and medication responses so much that you'll be faced with too much uncertainty to deal with safely.

10. Don't exercise if you have pain, numbness, or tingling in your feet. These could be signs of nerve damage or circulation problems that exercise could only make worse.

11. Drink lots of fluids. This is important for all exercisers, but those with diabetes especially. Drink before exercise, during exercise if it's longer than about 20 minutes, and afterward. Water generally is considered the best choice, but for exercise sessions lasting more than 30 minutes or so, a drink containing a small amount of carbohydrate (about 15 grams) may be advisable to help keep blood sugar levels in a safe range.

12. Eat enough after you've exercised. Blood sugar levels can continue to fall for as long as 24 hours after a vigorous or prolonged workout, so be sure to eat sufficiently—and monitor your glucose levels often—to be sure your food "tank" is being adequately refilled.

13. Don't exercise alone in isolated areas. This is especially true if you tend to suffer from low sugar, which could cause you to lose consciousness. If you must experience the great outdoors, take along a family member or friend.

14.   Carry a fast-acting carbohydrate snack. It doesn't have to be a basket lunch but rather just some raisins, a nondiet soda or sports beverage, some crackers, or a ready-made glucose gel or glucose tablets sold at pharmacies to come to your rescue should your blood sugar levels begin to fall too low.

15. Carry identification. In addition to specifying that you have diabetes and what type, this ID card should include your address, phone number, your physician's name and phone number, the name and number of someone to call in an emergency, and the dosages of insulin or other medications you use. It can be a good idea to carry change for a phone call or a cellular phone, too.

16. Keep on top of your feet. This means well-fitting shoes designed specifically for the activity you're doing: no jogging in tennis shoes or walking in dress shoes, please. It also means checking your feet every day for any signs of irritation such as blisters, redness, cuts, or open sores. Diabetes can make such conditions more dangerous than they would be for the average person, so keep close watch and report what might appear to be even just minor problems to your doctor to play it safe. (If you have any trouble checking the bottoms of your feet, use a handheld mirror.) Your feet are your primary exercise "wheels," remember, so it pays to keep them in good working order.

QUESTIONS TO ASK YOUR DOCTOR

Any advice on exercise given here should be considered quite general compared to the more specific recommendations you should get from your doctor, diabetes educator, or exercise specialist. Your case is as individual as you are, remember, and because exercise can have such profound effects on some of the most critical aspects of diabetes—

including how your body responds to medication—the exercise advice you receive should be as custom-tailored to your particular condition as possible.

With that in mind, be sure you do not begin your exercise efforts until you get these following questions answered by your doctor or members of your health care team:

- How often should I exercise?

- How strenuously should I exercise, and for how long? Are any times of the day better for me to exercise than others?

- Should I stick to the same exercise routine each day, or may I vary my activities?

- Should I monitor my exertion levels with a heart rate monitor?

- Are there any types of exercise I should avoid?

- Are there certain signs I should look for that could indicate danger such as chest pains or feeling light-headed or dizzy?

- Should I alter my insulin dosage or be careful of where I inject before exercising?

- How will I need to modify my eating schedule to accommodate my exercise?

- Will oral medications affect me differently if I exercise?

INTENSITY AND STRETCHING

What's the very best exercise program you can do?

Any exercise program that you in fact *will* do, the experts unanimously agree. If more of us had ignored the cries of "no pain, no gain" and "go for the burn" two decades ago, we might not be as ample as we are today. Millions of us threw in the towel before even making it to the showers, and for a reason as simple as human nature itself: We do better when motivated by pleasure than pain. Do *not* make the mistake (again?) of being defeated by your own zeal. You want to be exercising for the rest of your life, remember, so do yourself the favor of proceeding more like the tortoise than the hare.

As expressed by the ADA, "Your activity should get your heart pumping and blood flowing but not be so intense as to cause you shortness of breath, weakness or pain." This should hold true whether you're walking, jogging, cycling, or clipping the hedges. By getting uncomfortably out of breath, you're starving your body of oxygen, and that's not what aerobic exercise is all about. It's about infusing your body's cells with oxygen, and only by breathing freely can you do that.

> *Y*ou want to be exercising for the rest of your life, remember, so do yourself the favor of proceeding more like the tortoise than the hare.

Try as best you can to keep your efforts continuous, too, whether it's a standard exercise such as using a stationary bike or treadmill, or something less traditional such as yard work or mopping the kitchen floor. Stop if you get tired, of course, but if you can keep moving for periods of at least 10 minutes, you give your heart and circulatory system a better chance of getting into a strengthening rhythm and flow.

Is stretching necessary? Not so much for preventing injury if your activities are going to be relatively moderate, such as walking or doing light work around the house or yard. In preparation for more intense activities such as jogging or weight-lifting, however, yes, a light warm-up that includes gentle stretching is a good idea. As we get older, moreover, regular stretching in addition to our calorie-burning aerobic activities can be a good idea to prevent the shortening and tightening of muscles that tends to occur with age. Talk to your doctor, diabetes educator, or exercise specialist about some stretches suited for your needs. (Many people find yoga can be particularly helpful for combating the stiffness that can accompany our reconciliations with Father Time.)

Exercise for the Expecting

Does pregnancy present problems for the mom with diabetes who wants to stay fit?

Not if activities are done safely. Exercise can be helpful for controlling blood sugar levels—which is as important for your baby as it is for you—and it can give you the stamina you may need for delivery in addition to helping you maintain a healthy weight. You should check with your diabetes doctor as well as your obstetrician to come up with a program that's best for you, however, and you'll want to keep your workouts fairly light. You'll also want to be careful to avoid low blood sugar levels when exercising, which could mean testing your glucose seven or more times a day. Here are some other tips for keeping your exercise as safe and healthful as it can be:

- Work closely with your health care team to come up with a glucose monitoring schedule that will keep your blood sugar levels as stable as possible.

- Drink plenty of fluids before, during, and after your exercise sessions.

LOOK BEFORE YOU LEAP INTO A HEALTH CLUB

Should you join a health club or gym to help keep your exercise efforts on track?

That's a question only you can answer. If you're easily intimidated by the presence of other people who may be more fit than you, probably not. But if you think such folks may inspire you and you're the type who likes structure, it might be a good idea. A health club can be an especially good idea if you'd like to do strength training, which is best done with professional guidance and can require costly equipment to be done safely and well. Joining a club also can be a good way

- Take time to warm up before and cool down after your workouts.

- Keep the most strenuous part of your exercise session no longer than about 15 minutes.

- Try not to exceed a heart rate of about 140 beats per minute as you exercise (this will be about 23 beats for a 10-second count).

- Keep your body temperature under 100 degrees Fahrenheit, and don't use a hot tub or steam room without checking with your doctor.

- Stop exercising if you feel light-headed, weak, or unusually out of breath.

- Ask your obstetrician about how to check for uterine contractions during exercise—they could be a sign you're overdoing it.

- Avoid exercises that require you to lie on your back (after your 4th month), strain, hold your breath, or do movements that are jerky or require quick changes in direction.

to get an idea of some of the latest fitness devices available, should you decide to purchase a similar device for use at home. Whether it's a stationary bike, stair climber, elliptical trainer, or rowing machine, lighter-weight and less expensive models usually are available for home use.

You don't want to be losing your shirt instead of those unwanted pounds, however, so be sure to get the following issues straight before signing on any dotted lines:

- **What exactly will your membership include?** Expect a free fitness evaluation plus at least one session with an instructor to get you started on the program of your choice.

- **Can you get a refund if you suffer from a health problem or you decide to move?** If this is important to you and the answer is no, move on.

- **Can you use clubs in other cities if the club is part of a chain?** This can be a nice feature if you're a frequent traveler.

- **Can you get a discount by using the club during off hours?** Daytime weekday rates should be lower.

- **What qualifications do the instructors have?** You can call the American Council on Exercise at (800) 529-8227 to get the full scoop on what to look for.

Still Sedentary After All These Years

Despite all the proven benefits of exercise, only about one in five Americans currently gets the amount necessary for cashing in on these rewards, according a recent *Journal of the American Medical Association* report. Why our reluctance to partake?

It's a great question, but not one with some very good answers, unfortunately. The President's Council on Physical Fitness and Sports did a nationwide survey recently to find out our major excuses for not being more physically active, and here are the ones cited most often. How many might you be guilty of?

"I don't have enough time." This was the most common excuse, cited by 40 percent of respondents, yet it may be the least legitimate of all given that our leisure time is at an all-time high.

"I get enough exercise at work or around the house." This was cited by 20 percent of respondents, but it also must be considered suspect given that our current rates of obesity also are higher than they've ever been.

"I have health problems preventing me from exercising." This one might more accurately be, "I have health problems be-

- **Is the club's equipment leased or owned?** Leased is better because the equipment will tend to be more up-to-date.

Remember, too, that if you yearn for the structure or exercise gadgetry but money is an issue, you can always check out your local YMCA, community center, or college gym.

DON'T FORGET THE KIDS

As you're doing what you can to turn your own exercise life around, don't forget the family. Studies show that 40 percent of American

---

cause I don't exercise." Next to not smoking, exercise has been shown to be the single most effective thing we can do to help prevent many of the most serious and chronic health problems we face today.

"Exercise is too boring." Sorry, but in light of the new "anything goes" exercise guidelines, people using this excuse are admitting that what, in fact, must be boring is them.

"I'm too old to exercise." This is more fitting as an epitaph than an excuse. Studies show that we can derive huge benefits from exercise even well into our 90s.

"I'm too tired to exercise." Sorry, but research shows that exercise can do more to cure fatigue than cause it. No points here.

"Exercise isn't necessary." For anyone who doesn't care about how long they live, maybe not. Some studies, however, indicate that greater exercise participation in the United States could prevent as many as 250,000 early deaths a year.

New Fitness Credos

Tired of the old rallying cry of "no pain, no gain"? Join the club. Here are some fitness credos that many of us might do well to put on our refrigerator doors:

"Pleasure is better at burning calories than pain."

"Exercise is like money in the bank: Every calorie counts."

"You're too busy to exercise only if you're too busy to breathe."

"Those aren't stairs—they're steps to a longer life!"

"Weed the garden; harvest your health."

"Cut the grass and your risks of heart disease, too."

"Go for the trees and the forest will come."

children have the makings of heart disease (including obesity, high blood pressure, and high blood fats) well underway by the age of 8! Research also shows that two-thirds of children between the ages of 6 and 16 can't pass standard fitness tests given in school and that three-quarters of children who are obese as adolescents (a figure that's at an all-time high) go on to be obese as adults.

It's not a comforting picture, and it's one that's up to *us* as both parents and role models to do what we can to change. Setting a good example with our own exercise programs is good for starters, of course, but many experts suggest we go a step further by actually including our children in our exercise efforts whenever possible—for example, on walks, in sporting activities, on bike rides, or with chores around the house or yard. We can join them on their turf, too, going to the playground or playing jump rope, hopscotch, dodgeball, or hide-and-seek. It's amazing the muscle groups these "childish" activities can get to and the full-body workouts they can give.

Then, too, we can address what steals the activity from our children in the first place—the national average of 25 hours of TV a week, the computer games, the junk food, and weekends spent watching movies from the video store. A mind is a terrible thing to waste, and a body is, too.

THE PROS AND CONS OF MORE VIGOROUS EXERCISE

The new "kinder and gentler" approach to exercise is great because it can welcome less athletic types into the fitness family, but this is not to say that more regimented or strenuous types of exercise such as jogging or working out on stationary bikes or rowing machines need to be avoided. With your doctor's approval and supervision and with appropriate instruction on glucose monitoring and adjustments to medication and meal planning you may need to make, vigorous activity can be even more potent medicine for controlling blood sugar than a more moderate approach. The reason is very simple: The more vigorous an activity is, the more calories it burns, and these calories come primarily from glucose. In addition to helping to control blood sugar levels, this greater calorie burn can be a plus for weight control as well.

With your doctor's approval and supervision and with appropriate instruction, vigorous activity can be even more potent medicine for controlling blood sugar than a more moderate approach.

Something to be aware of, however, if you plan to give vigorous forms of exercise a try: Glucose levels in the blood may actually rise in the beginning stages of such activities, because certain stress hormones cued by vigorous exercise will cause your body to mobilize blood sugar stored in your liver to help provide the required fuel. If there is not enough insulin in your system (either injected insulin or your body's own) to escort this glucose into the exercising muscles, blood sugar levels could continue to rise, thus defeating the purpose of the exercise in addition to risking the dangerous state of ketoacidosis, in which the body has no choice but to derive its energy solely from fat.

Consider it critical, therefore, to get the okay from your doctor in addition to special instruction on medication levels and glucose monitoring before giving the following vigorous forms of exercise a try. This point shouldn't discourage you but rather only encourage you to do what's necessary to keep these activities as safe and beneficial as possible.

Jogging. A fantastic calorie burner and fitness builder, but it can be tough on weight-bearing joints, the feet, and the lower back for people with disc problems.

Cycling (outdoor as well as stationary). Also a great calorie-burning fitness activity, with the advantage of being easy on weight-bearing joints, the feet, and back.

Swimming. A great full-body exercise, easy on the joints, and especially good for people with arthritis or back trouble.

Rowing. Another great full-body workout, although potentially aggravating for low back pain.

Brisk walking. All things considered, possibly the best all-around fitness activity we have—safe, enjoyable, and practical in that it can get us places we need to go without necessarily requiring special workout clothes or a shower. Carrying weights while walking can give the arms a good workout, too.

ANNE PETERS—THE MIND (AND HEART) BEHIND THE MIRACLE

She wasn't there at his side at the medal ceremonies, but she should have been—Anne Peters, M.D., the brains behind the brawn that accomplished what many thought would be impossible. Three other doctors had told Gary Hall that with type 1 diabetes, his chances of swimming competitively at the Olympic level were as good as the snowball in you know where. But Gary wouldn't hear it, so he found himself the doctor that would share his "insanity"—and turn it into Olympic gold.

Despite having her hands full as the director of Clinical Diabetes at the University of Southern California Keck School of Medicine, Dr. Peters devoted herself to working meticulously with Gary to fine-tune every aspect of his treatment, including medication, glucose monitoring, and diet. She was there at poolside with him when he trained, helping him with his monitoring, advising him when to "pull over" during his longer swims to snack, and counseling him on how to eat after his grueling workouts to gain the strength his marathon effort was going to require. To let Gary prove he could be the best of the best—despite his metabolic "disadvantage"—was going to take a marathon of her own, but she welcomed the challenge every bit as much as the man in the pool.

"I saw in Gary someone who would do whatever it took to win, and not just for himself but for others," Dr. Peters says. "He wanted to succeed to show other diabetics that they could succeed, too, that diabetes doesn't have to get in the way of anything, no matter how impossible it might seem."

So doctor and patient worked as partners, fine-tuning what would have to be a near-perfect athletic machine to succeed against the very best in the world. "Gary was the driving force, though," Dr. Peters says. "And this is the way it should be with diabetes," she adds. "It's the patient who ultimately needs to take charge of treatment because only the patient can know what really works. Gary listened to my advice, of course, but he also made changes that he found worked best for him. He learned about his disease, and he paid close attention to his diet and close attention to his body, monitoring his glucose as often as 10 times a day. He worked incredibly hard to make his treatment work."

Gary is the first to give the credit for his success to Dr. Peters, but the way she sees it, the credit should go to him. "Sure, I helped, but he's the one who did the work and provided the all-important feedback so that we could work as a team," she says. "That's the key to overcoming this disease, I'm convinced—for physicians and patients to work together as closely as possible. Every case is just so different that treatment has to be worked out day-to-day, often through trial and error, until the best solutions are found. I don't know of any other disease that requires doctor and patients to work together so closely as a team."

> *That's the key to overcoming this disease, I'm convinced—for physicians and patients to work together as closely as possible.*

But then that's why Dr. Peters chose the field of diabetes, she says. "I know it sounds corny, but I wanted to be able to make a difference in people's lives, both as a scientist and as a person. And diabetes has certainly let me do that. What I've found is that one heals by applying not just the best technology but also good old-fashioned love. We've got to show compassion and do more to encourage our patients to get involved in their own treatment the way Gary did. The best medicine is a healing partnership."

And this is as true at home as it is at the hospital, Dr. Peters says. "Diabetes is a very demanding disease that requires support and love from everyone associated with it. The family members and friends of patients often can go through as much as the patients themselves, and these people need to know just how important they are.

"Every person with diabetes faces the same challenge as Gary in a way, and that's to be the very best they can," Dr. Peters adds. "There might not be gold medals waiting for them when they succeed, but there certainly should be. What they're succeeding at, after all, is the greatest goal of all—to live a full and meaningful life."

CHAPTER 7

Complementary Treatments

Nature's Best Shots

❧

W HEN A DISEASE is as widespread as diabetes (affecting approximately 1 in 17 Americans) and as wide-ranging in its effects (virtually every major organ suffers in some way), it should come as no surprise that a wide variety of health practitioners are going to want to try their healing hands. Therapists ranging from herbalists to acupuncturists in recent years have been taking their best shots.

But with what success? That's what this chapter is about. And at the risk of spoiling its ending, we'll say up-front that although the kind of proof that mainstream medicine likes to see might not always be there, reason to feel encouraged most certainly is. Speaking at the American Diabetes Association's 60th Annual Scientific Sessions, for example, Laura McWhorter, Pharm.D., an associate professor and certified diabetes educator at the University of Utah School of Medicine, advised that physicians begin taking a closer look at the treatment benefits that certain herbs and nutritional supplements may have to offer. For day-to-day control of glucose level as well as treating long-term complications of diabetes, Dr. McWhorter reported, these "complementary" treatments should not be overlooked.

Dr. McWhorter's announcement might be viewed as more icing on the cake for complementary medicine in general, which has been gaining respect not just from patients in recent years but also from the traditional Western (allopathic) medical system. Complementary medical practitioners now attract more visits and out-of-pocket payment from patients each year than medicine of conventional Western origin. Forty-two percent of Americans now regularly utilize an alternative medical therapy of some type and spend over $21 billion a year in doing so, according to a recent *Journal of the American Medical Association* report. Our use of herbs has increased by nearly fourfold in the past decade alone, for example, and our use of nutritional supplements in this time has nearly doubled.

> *Complementary medical practitioners now attract more visits and out-of-pocket payment from patients each year than medicine of conventional Western origin.*

Are we getting results? To what degree we've been healing ourselves with our own placebo effects when using alternative therapies is hard to say because the modalities are just now beginning to undergo well-controlled scientific evaluation (see "What to Look for in a Study"). We do know that millions of patients are finding satisfaction with many of these alternative therapies, however. Besides, more than 75 medical schools in the United States now offer training in one or more alternative medical practices, and a growing number of physicians have started adding some form of alternative therapy to widen the scope and appeal of their traditional lineup of treatments. The "renegade" therapies must be doing something right.

With respect to diabetes, let's see what that is.

WHAT TO LOOK FOR IN A STUDY

As you read through the medical evidence in this chapter, it can be helpful to know what makes the results of some research studies more meaningful than others. A complaint against many of the claims made

A Note of Caution: Complement, Don't Replace

Although many alternative healing therapies could be said to be "natural," this descriptor does not assure that they're always safe, especially when a disease as potentially serious as diabetes is involved. Consider it of utmost importance, therefore, that you continue your normal care with your health care team and that you keep them informed of all aspects of the alternative treatments you plan to pursue. If you're considering herbs or nutritional supplements, for example, be sure to let your doctor know exactly what you intend to try because some of these remedies could affect the pharmaceutical actions of certain diabetes medications.

The word the medical community has adopted to characterize alternative healing techniques is *complementary*, remember—a word chosen for a reason. Your alternative healing efforts should complement your conventional medical care, not replace it.

by alternative healing techniques in general, in fact, is that the supporting research is not always as scientifically sound as experts would like.

Here, therefore, are the key features to look for as you peruse the following findings. The more of these standards that a particular study satisfies, the more valid and hence important its conclusions are apt to be. The most respected scientific investigations are those with the following qualities:

- **Large**. Yes, bigger is better. The more people a study involves, the less the potential for error due to chance. As you read through the following reports, therefore, consider the results of a study involving 1,200 people to be worth significantly more attention than one involving 12.

- **Conducted with human subjects.** For convenience as well as safety, studies sometimes are done under laboratory conditions involving test tubes and petri dishes rather than with real people. While more convenient, such studies are not generally deemed to be as reliable as those involving real human beings or laboratory animals.

- **Well controlled.** The best studies are those that compare the results of giving a "real" treatment to one group of people against the results of giving a "fake" treatment (a placebo) to another. Also important is that the study be conducted in what's called a *double-blind* fashion, meaning neither the researchers nor the people being tested know to whom the real treatment is being given. The purpose of this is to eliminate as much as possible what's known as the *placebo effect*, whereby test subjects will display the suspected result due purely to psychological influence.

So be savvy and keep these criteria in mind as you assess the often intriguing if not always highly significant research reports discussed in this chapter. Much of the research being done on herbs and nutritional supplements in the United States is still in its infant stages, unfortunately. The Europeans are far ahead of us in this area, but you may trust that American researchers are trying to catch up as fast as good science will allow.

Finally, if you have questions about the reliability or safety of any product touted as a diabetes remedy, you can check with the American Diabetes Association to get its official opinion by calling (800) 342-2383. The ADA regularly reviews such products and places them in one of four categories based on its findings:

- Clearly effective
- Somewhat or sometimes effective for certain types of patients
- Unknown or unproven but possibly promising
- Clearly ineffective

HERBS AGAINST HIGH BLOOD SUGAR

Many of the herbs discussed here have been used to treat diabetes for thousands of years in India and China but have not come under the scrutiny of modern science until fairly recently, unfortunately. Even these studies have been done mostly in India, moreover, where these herbs have been of greater importance in the medical system. We should regard these findings accordingly but have reason to consider them encouraging, nonetheless.

Note: It's important to keep in mind that if any of these treatments proves effective, you will need to reduce whatever medication you may be taking to avoid hypoglycemia. For this reason, you should not be trying these treatments without the supervision of your doctor or health care team.

Gymnema (*Gymnema sylvestre*)

The use of this herb for treating diabetes in India goes back more than 2,000 years, and research into its effectiveness for treating both types 1 and 2 have been underway since the 1930s. None of the studies has been double-blind, unfortunately, but results might be viewed as intriguing. In one study of people with type 1 diabetes, 27 patients were given (in addition to their usual insulin) 400 milligrams a day of *Gymnema sylvestre* for 6 to 30 months, while another group of 37 patients continued their standard insulin therapy alone. Results were impressive: The herb group was able to decrease insulin needs by 50 percent as their average glucose levels dropped by 80 points from 232 to 152 milligrams/deciliter. Their glycosylated hemoglobin (HbA1c) also dropped significantly after 6 to 8 months of taking the herb, while the control group showed no significant improvements at all.

Researchers doing the type 1 study also conducted a similar trial on type 2 patients and with similarly encouraging results. The same dosage, 400 milligrams daily, was given (in conjunction with their oral medications) to 22 patients with type 2 diabetes for 18 to 20 months, and sure enough—the group experienced lower glucose levels as well

ver glycosylated hemoglobin, and their pancreatic release of in-
ncreased as well. This allowed the group as a whole to reduce
oral medication, while 5 of the 22 patients were able to discontinue
their drugs entirely.

> **How it might work.** Subsequent studies with *Gymnema* using
> animals have shown that the herb may help regenerate insulin-
> secreting cells in the pancreas while also inhibiting glucose ab-
> sorption in the intestines and increasing glucose absorption by
> the cells.

> **Safety.** No serious adverse reactions have been found to occur
> with this herb, but its safety has not been established for peo-
> ple with liver or kidney damage or for pregnant or nursing
> women. Because it may lower blood sugar levels, moreover, it
> should not be used without medical supervision.

> **Recommended dosage.** *Gymnema sylvestre* is sold in extract
> form standardized to 24 percent gymnemic acid, with the rec-
> ommended dosage being between 400 and 600 milligrams a day.

Bitter Lemon (*Momordica charantia*)

Also known as balsam pear or bitter gourd, this herb has a long history of use against diabetes in China and is thought to house its most
medicinally active compound—*p-insulin*—in its fruit and seeds. This
compound closely resembles insulin derived from cows in its molecular structure; not surprisingly, it has been found to function much like
bovine insulin when injected into patients with type 1 diabetes.

Studies of this herb are limited by not being double-blind in design, but they still have produced intriguing results. In one study, 90
out of 100 people newly diagnosed with type 2 diabetes experienced
significant drops in their blood sugar when they drank 100 milliliters
(about 1/2 cup) of juice made from the bitter lemon fruit. In another
study that looked at the effects of bitter lemon on blood sugar levels
over time, a 100-milliliter drink made from an extract of the herb
lowered glucose levels in seven people with type 2 diabetes by an av-

erage of 54 percent after 3 weeks; after 7 weeks, a significant drop in glycosylated hemoglobin was observed.

How it might work. Studies with animals suggest that bitter lemon works to lower glucose levels by increasing glucose uptake by the cells.

Safety. The safety of bitter lemon has not been proven in formal studies, but its use in a variety of forms throughout much of Asia for centuries suggests it poses no unusual risks. As with most herbs, however, pregnant or nursing women should not use bitter lemon, nor should young children or anyone with liver or kidney disease.

Recommended dosage. Dosage depends on the form in which bitter lemon is taken. If taken as juice made fresh from the fruit (which you should be warned is extremely bitter, however), daily dosage is generally between 50 and 100 milliliters ($^1/_4$ to $^1/_2$ cup). Easier on the taste buds is to take capsules that contain dried powder made from the fruit, with the standard dose being between three and fifteen 1-gram capsules daily. For ease of use, however, most herbalists recommend taking bitter lemon as a standardized extract according to instructions on the label—usually in the range of 100 to 200 milligrams three times daily.

Fenugreek (*Trigonella foenum graecum*)

Most people are familiar with this herb more for its culinary talents than its medicinal might, but that could soon change as its effects on blood sugar become better known. Fenugreek seeds contain its active component, which has been shown to lower glucose levels in people with type 1 and type 2 diabetes alike. In one controlled study involving ten people with type 1 diabetes, five were given 50 grams of defatted fenugreek seed powder twice daily with lunch and dinner, while the other patients were not. After 10 days, the fenugreek group showed lower glucose in their blood and urine, as well as reductions in serum cholesterol.

Other studies, although not double-blind, have replicated these results in type 2 diabetics, and with lower doses. In one, just 25 grams of fenugreek daily resulted in improvements in glucose control, glucose elevations in response to a meal, and the amount of glucose in the urine. Another study obtained similar results with just 15 grams daily, and many studies done with animals have confirmed fenugreek's glucose-reducing talents.

How it might work. Scientists think fenugreek may work in the same way as drugs known as alpha-glucosidase inhibitors, which help keep blood sugar levels down by interfering with glucose absorption in the intestines, though much still needs to be learned.

Safety. Anecdotal evidence suggests fenugreek may interfere with the absorption of oral diabetes medications. Although this has not been confirmed by formal research, most experts suggest patients separate taking fenugreek and oral diabetic agents by at least 2 hours. High dosages also may cause mild gastrointestinal discomfort, and the herb should not be used (in dosages higher than those commonly used in cooking) by pregnant or nursing women, young children, or people with liver or kidney disease.

Recommended dosage. Because the seeds of fenugreek can be somewhat bitter, most herbalists recommend taking the herb in capsule form, with a typical dose being 5 to 30 grams taken three times a day with meals. The herb is also available in powder form, which can be mixed with foods, beverages, or shakes to add a nutty flavor.

Asian and American Ginseng (*Panax ginseng* and *Panax quinquefolius*)

Already on record for being an energizer, these two types of ginseng (but not Siberian ginseng, which is not truly ginseng at all) appear to be helpful in treating type 2 diabetes. In one recent double-blind study, 36 people newly diagnosed with type 2 diabetes experienced lower glucose levels as well as more physical energy after being given Asian ginseng for 8 weeks. Similar results were observed in two smaller, double-blind, and placebo-controlled studies using American ginseng.

How it might work. The actions of ginseng are not well understood, but some researchers speculate that reductions in blood sugar could result from the increases in physical activity that the herb tends to spur.

Safety. Side effects from ginseng are rare, although women sometimes report menstrual irregularities or breast tenderness. Some reports suggest ginseng may interact with certain prescription drugs, however—MAO inhibitors and blood thinners, for example—so be sure to check with your doctor if you're taking either of these. Also know that ginseng's safety has not been confirmed for pregnant or nursing women, young children, or people with liver or kidney disease.

Recommended dosage. The typical daily dose of Asian ginseng is 1 to 2 grams of the raw herb, or 200 milligrams of an extract standardized to contain 4 to 7 percent ginsenosides. In the study mentioned using American ginseng, 3 grams daily were used.

OTHER HERBS SHOWING PROMISE FOR GLUCOSE CONTROL

Because fewer studies have been done on these following herbs, we can give no recommended dosages. Research has shown that they can have a positive impact on glucose control, however, so they may be worth looking into with the help of a qualified herbalist who may have experience in working with them. As with most herbs, however, these should not be tried without medical supervision, and their safety has not been confirmed for pregnant or nursing women or people with liver or kidney disease.

Aloe vera. Yes, the gel that's become so popular for treating cuts and burns from the outside seems to have good things in store for people with diabetes when taken internally. In one recent placebo-controlled study, for example, people with type 2 diabetes given 1 tablespoon of *Aloe vera* juice twice daily for 2 weeks showed significantly lower blood sugar levels than patients not given the herb. Another placebo-controlled study showed that a similar dosage of aloe, given in conjunction with the oral medication glibenclamide, was helpful in lowering glucose levels in type 2 patients who had not been responding to glibenclamide alone.

Bilberry (*Vaccinium myrtillus*). This botanical cousin of the blueberry (which also has talents for helping prevent certain complications of diabetes, as we'll be seeing shortly) has been shown in animal studies to lower not just blood sugar but also triglycerides, making it helpful in combating heart disease. Eaten as fruit, bilberry has been shown to be safe, but it's safety has not been confirmed for pregnant or nursing women or people with liver or kidney disease when taken as an extract.

Coccinia indica. In one double-blind study that involved 32 patients for a period of 6 weeks, 16 of whom were given a preparation made from the leaves of this herb daily, 10 of those 16 experienced marked improvement in blood sugar control, while no such improvement was seen in any of the control group of 16 patients who received a placebo instead. Studies done with animals suggest the herb may work by increasing glucose uptake by the cells.

Holy basil (*Ocimum sanctum* and *Ocimum album*). A group of 40 people with type 2 diabetes experienced reductions in blood sugar when they were given a preparation made from holy basil leaves for 4 weeks, but they experienced no such reductions during a 4-week period in which they were given a placebo.

Pterocarpus marsupium. A study done in India found that this herb, in dosages between 2 and 4 grams daily, helped 67 out of 97 type 2 patients attain better blood sugar control after 12 weeks, results supported by test tube research as well as studies with animals. Other studies done with extracts of this herb found that it helped protect beta (insulin-producing) cells in animals given diabetes-causing substances.

CAN CERTAIN FOODS FIGHT HIGH BLOOD SUGAR?

The research is preliminary, but yes, it seems that some foods contain compounds that may help keep blood sugar levels under control. Onions and garlic, for example, contain substances that appear to slow the rise of blood sugar following a meal, possibly by interfering with the way the liver normally deactivates insulin, some studies suggest. Given the safety of these foods, not to mention their talents for giving meals added pizzazz, it certainly couldn't hurt to incorporate them whenever possible into your meals.

The same is true for the Jerusalem artichoke, which contains a substance known as *inulin* that some research suggests may retard the usual rise in blood sugar following a meal by slowing the absorption of glucose by the intestines. Also an excellent source of fiber, folate, vitamin C, and magnesium—while being low in calories and virtually fat-free—the artichoke is a food to be taken to heart. Burdock root and dandelion are two other edible inulin sources.

BEST NUTRIENTS FOR KEEPING GLUCOSE IN LINE

Just as research has been showing that certain herbs may be able to aid the quest for better glucose control, studies are finding that certain nutrients may also have promise—the trace mineral chromium, for example, plus certain B vitamins and magnesium. Exceptionally high dosages of these nutrients usually have been required to produce positive results, however, so while the nutrients themselves may be natural, the amounts needed to achieve medicinal effects are not. Risks for adverse side effects from these nutrients also increase as dosages rise, so while encouraging, the potential benefits of these nutrients also must be viewed with these drawbacks in mind.

As we'll be seeing, some nutritional supplements can actually be detrimental for blood sugar control, so clearly a substance should not be judged as universally benign just because it's derived from a food. And as always, don't even think about trying a nutritional supplement or any complementary treatment for diabetes without discussing your plans with your diabetes educator or doctor.

Chromium

The human need for this trace mineral, which the body requires for metabolizing sugar and fat, wasn't even known to scientists until 1977 when patients who were getting no chromium at all in their diets (as a result of being fed intravenously in a hospital setting) were found to develop diabetes. Subsequent studies went on to discover that while the mineral is required in only very small amounts—between 50 and 200 micrograms daily—most Americans get only about 30 micrograms in their diets. This shortage is compounded by the fact that diabetes limits absorption of the mineral and by the fact that foods high in sugar and refined white flour tend to do the same.

But can chromium help lower blood sugar levels in diabetics? Deficiencies aside, this is the question that continues to be argued today, and which the following studies have addressed. In one double-blind study done in 1997, 180 people with type 2 diabetes were divided into three groups: one receiving 500 micrograms of chromium twice daily, another getting 100 micrograms twice daily, and the third being given a placebo containing no chromium at all. After 4 months, during which the patients continued their normal diabetes treatments, the highest-dosage chromium group showed significantly lower fasting glucose levels, while no changes were seen in the other two groups. Also measured, however, were glycosylated hemoglobin levels—the long-term method of glucose surveillance—and in this respect, both chromium groups showed improvement (the high-dosage group more so than the lower-dosage patients), while the placebo group showed no change at all. The high-dosage group showed glycosylated hemoglobin levels that were normal, in fact, while they were the only group to show lower cholesterol levels as well.

Not all studies done with chromium have produced such positive results, however, and some have shown no results at all. In the words of alternative medicine expert Steven Bratman, M.D., the author of several books on the alternative medicine movement, "In the case of chromium, the balance of evidence appears to suggest that supplementation can be helpful." Dr. Bratman adds that of the various forms of chromium available, chromium picolinate and chromium citrate have been shown to be the best absorbed.

> **How it might work.** The precise biochemical mechanisms behind chromium's effects on blood sugar are not fully understood, but scientists speculate that the mineral may work, at least in part, by helping insulin bind to receptor cites on the body's cells, thus decreasing insulin resistance and facilitating glucose uptake.

> **Safety.** Safety, unfortunately, is where some experts feel chromium falls short of being suitable for widespread use; to be effective, the mineral needs to be used in amounts that some evidence suggests may pose considerable risks. The Estimated Safe and Adequate Daily Dietary Intake (ESADDI) of chromium established by the U.S. government, for example, has been put at 200 micrograms per day, yet the dosages shown to be effective at lowering blood sugar are in the range of five times that much. Any thought of trying chromium in potentially therapeutic

dosages, therefore, definitely needs to be discussed with your doctor.

While it may be true that the Environmental Protection Agency has put a limit on chromium exposure that exceeds the ESADDI standard by 350-fold, and animal studies have shown no toxic effects at levels 5,000 times higher than the ESADDI mark, toxicity in lesser amounts in humans has been reported. One case has been noted, for example, of a woman who began developing anemia, reduction in blood platelets, weight loss, and signs of liver and kidney damage after just 4 months of taking 1,200 to 2,400 micrograms of chromium (as chromium picolinate) daily. Speaking at the 60th Annual Scientific Sessions of the American Diabetes Association, moreover, Dr. McWhorter warned that other reported side effects from chromium use have included the eye disorder miosis, allergic skin reactions, and intensification of existing psychiatric disorders. Discuss all of these potential complications with your doctor before even considering giving chromium a try.

Best food sources. Brewer's yeast, brown rice, broccoli, potatoes, whole wheat products, ham, liver, and grape juice.

Recommended daily value. No recommended daily value has yet been established for chromium, but levels of between 50 and 200 micrograms daily are thought to be required.

Biotin

Biotin is one of the B-complex vitamins, which in amounts of about 300 micrograms daily (the current recommended daily value) helps the body metabolize carbohydrates, proteins, and fats. But increase this amount by about thirty- to sixtyfold to 8 to 16 grams a day, and some research indicates biotin can help people with type 1 and type 2 diabetes lower their blood sugar. Only two studies using such amounts have been done with humans so far, and although the results were en-

---

The Chromium-Insulin Conundrum

In support of the scientific evidence that chromium may be helpful in reducing blood sugar levels for people with type 2 diabetes is this biochemical conundrum: Studies show that chromium deficiencies may cause an increased need for insulin, while the high insulin levels characteristic of many cases of type 2 diabetes, in turn, have been shown to increase risks for chromium deficiency. Insulin, the "cure," in other words, might be looked at as part of chromium deficiency, the "problem." By supplementing with chromium, therefore, some researchers feel it might be possible to reduce needs for insulin—and in so doing also help "fix" what's causing chromium to be in short supply in the first place.

---

couraging, the studies were small as well as short in duration, so clearly more research with biotin needs to be done.

Researchers remain optimistic, however, because as a water-soluble vitamin, biotin does not accumulate in the body and hence has a low potential for causing for toxic effects even in high dosages. Some studies have shown that people with diabetes tend to be deficient in biotin, moreover, suggesting that supplementation may a good idea based on that alone.

How it might work. Biotin is thought to help lower blood sugar by improving insulin sensitivity while also stimulating the activity of an enzyme called *glucokinase* known to play a role in glucose uptake by the liver.

Safety. As mentioned, health risks associated with even very high does of biotin appear not to be a problem because excesses of this water-soluble vitamin simply leave the body via the urine.

Best food sources. Brewer's yeast, corn, barley, peanuts, soybeans, walnuts, liver, chicken, egg yolks, cauliflower, mushrooms, fortified cereals, and milk.

Recommended daily value. 300 micrograms.

Magnesium

Magnesium is involved in every major biological function—including helping insulin get glucose into the body's cells—but studies show that many people with diabetes tend to be deficient in this important mineral. Whether the shortage is due to problems with absorbing the mineral or losses of magnesium through excessive urination, doctors aren't sure yet, but they have learned that magnesium supplementation (above the current recommended daily value of 400 milligrams) may help control high blood sugar levels as well as minimize certain complications such as eye damage (retinopathy) commonly associated with the disease.

In one small, double-blind study done with eight elderly patients with type 2 diabetes, for example, 4 weeks of magnesium supplementation (2 grams daily) produced significantly improved insulin sensitivity and glucose uptake compared to another 4-week period during which the same people were given a placebo. In another study using dosages only about one-quarter as large (450 milligrams of magnesium daily), type 2 patients were found to produce more insulin, as well as clear blood sugar from their systems faster than before being given the mineral.

How it might work. Because magnesium is an important "catalyst" in so many vital biochemical reactions, scientists speculate that enhancing the activity of insulin may be one of them.

Safety. High dosages of magnesium (more than about 500 milligrams daily) have been associated with diarrhea in many people, and high dosages also should be avoided by people with kidney disease as well as pregnant and nursing women.

Best food sources. Brown rice, avocados, spinach, haddock, oatmeal, baked potatoes, beans, broccoli, yogurt, bananas, tofu, and apples.

Recommended daily value. 400 milligrams.

NUTRIENTS THAT MAY INTERFERE WITH GLUCOSE CONTROL

As proof of just how potent nutrients can be, research shows that large dosages of some dietary supplements can actually have adverse effects on blood sugar control, so be sure to check with your doctor if you're currently taking any of the supplements discussed here.

Iron

For a small number of people with diabetes, high levels of iron in the blood might actually be contributing to their disease, some research suggests, so you might want to have your doctor check your iron levels to play it safe. In one study of nine type 2 patients found to have elevated iron levels, eight of the patients who took a drug that cleared the excess iron from their systems experienced not only lower blood sugar but lower cholesterol and triglyceride levels as well.

Zinc

While deficiencies in zinc have been associated with making diabetes worse (by decreasing sensitivity to insulin), it seems too much of the mineral also may have adverse effects. One study found that people with type 1 diabetes experienced marked increases in blood sugar levels after taking 50 milligrams of zinc for 28 days, while another found that people with type 2 diabetes who took 270 milligrams of zinc (90 milligrams, three times daily) saw their fasting blood sugar levels rise by an average of about 15 percent from 177 to 207 milligrams/deciliter. If you're currently taking more than the recommended daily value of zinc—which is 15 milligrams—you should monitor your blood sugar carefully to be sure it's not having an adverse effect.

Glucosamine Sulfate

Helpful as this compound may be for treating and preventing wear and tear of the joints, recent research with animals as well anecdotal reports from humans suggest it may impair glucose tolerance and hence lead to higher blood sugar levels in people with diabetes. It also may increase risks of certain long-term complications of diabetes such as cataracts, so definitely check with your doctor if you're currently taking or are thinking about taking glucosamine sulfate supplements. By closely monitoring your blood sugar levels, you may be able to determine whether the supplementation is having any undesirable effects.

PREVENTING COMPLICATIONS WITH NATURE'S HELP

The war against diabetes can require more than just blood sugar control. Steps to minimize complications of the disease also can be worthwhile, and certain natural approaches may be able to lend a hand here, too. As always, though, you shouldn't attempt any complementary treatment without checking first with your doctor. Many of these remedies still are in the process of being tested for efficacy as well as safety, and their effects can vary from patient to patient, so you'll need to monitor your glucose closely and also keep watch for any adverse reactions. We'll start by looking at the natural remedies that are showing the most promise for diabetic neuropathy (nerve damage), then move on to eye problems, and finally examine heart and kidney complications.

Natural Protection for the Nerves

Neuropathy, as you may recall from chapter 1, refers to the nerve damage that consistently elevated blood sugar levels can cause, and it can occur in the nerves that are under voluntary (such as those in the arms and legs) as well as involuntary (such as those in the heart, stomach, and blood vessels) control. Some research in recent years has given hope that certain nutritional supplements may help thwart this potentially crippling consequence of diabetes, however. Because neuropathy takes years to develop, researchers have not been able to prove definitively that these nutritional aids can help halt diabetic nerve damage, but based on the following evidence, optimism is certainly in order. These nutrients are thought to exert their protective effects in one or more of the following ways:

- By helping prevent swelling of nerve cells caused by the conversion of glucose within the cells into a substance known as *sorbitol*, which attracts water

- By helping maintain normal levels of a compound important for healthy nerve function called *inositol*

- By inhibiting damage to fat molecules within nerve cells caused by naturally occurring molecular misfits known as *free radicals*

- By helping maintain proper blood flow and hence keeping nerve cells adequately nourished

Gamma-Linolenic Acid

Don't let the ominous-sounding name throw you. Gamma-linolenic acid (GLA) is a type of essential fatty acid (EFA) similar to the healthful fats found in cold-water fish. People without diabetes are able to make GLA from linoleic acid, a type of unsaturated fat common in many vegetable oils, but some research shows that diabetes seems to disrupt this process, making GLA supplementation advisable.

GLA has been shown to be important not just for helping to treat diabetic nerve damage, moreover: Adequate amounts are needed to prevent dry skin, hair loss, immune deficiency, and possibly arthritis, so it's not a nutrient to be slighted. With respect to neuropathy, one double-blind study of 111 patients found that those receiving

480 milligrams of GLA daily for a period of a year showed significant improvement over a placebo group in 13 out of 16 tests designed to measure the severity of nerve damage symptoms. Similar results were obtained by another placebo-controlled study in which patients were given 360 milligrams of GLA daily in the form of primrose oil for 6 months.

Note: Other studies done with animals suggest that GLA may be even more effective in controlling symptoms of diabetic nerve damage when taken in combination with alpha-lipoic acid, discussed next.

How it might work. GLA appears to protect nerves from damage by increasing blood flow and thus helping keep nerve cells well nourished with oxygen and other vital nutrients.

Safety. The safety of GLA has been well studied and well confirmed. The only reported problems—and in fewer than 2 percent of all users—have been complaints of headaches or mild gastrointestinal distress.

Therapeutic dosages. In the studies mentioned, dosages ranged from 360 to 480 milligrams of GLA daily—the amount in about 4 to 5 grams of primrose oil, which has a GLA concentration of 9 percent. Other sources of GLA—black currant oil or borage oil—may be used in lesser amounts because they contain 18 and 24 percent GLA, respectively. (All oils containing GLA should be stored in a dark cool place such as the refrigerator to avoid spoilage.)

Alpha-Lipoic Acid

Again, don't be put off by the decidedly synthetic-sounding name. This is a substance produced naturally in the body, and although test results have been mixed, it shows promise for treating diabetic neuropathy. The supplement appears to be more effective when injected, unfortunately, than when taken orally, and it suffers from the additional drawback of seeming to be effective only for about 3 weeks. These disadvantages in treating peripheral neuropathy aside, the nutrient does appear capable of reducing symptoms of autonomic (involuntary nerve) neuropathy, however, as evidenced by a double-blind study in which oral doses of 800 milligrams daily significantly improved irregular heartbeat in 29 diabetics after 4 months.

How it might work. Both test tube and animal studies suggest that alpha-lipoic acid may come at the problem of diabetic neuropathy from several angles. As an antioxidant it has been shown to reduce damage to nerve cells caused by free radicals, but it also reduces sorbitol accumulation (and hence swelling) within nerve cells while increasing blood flow.

Safety. Although formal safety studies have not been completed, no serious side effects from alpha-lipoic acid have been reported during its many years of use in Germany. Because high doses of alpha-lipoic acid have been found to be toxic to rats deficient in thiamin (vitamin B_1), however, some herbalists suggest accompanying the use of alpha-lipoic acid with 50 milligrams of this B vitamin daily. It also can be a good idea to check your blood sugar levels regularly if using this supplement because cases of hypoglycemia have been reported as a result of its glucose-lowering effects. As with most herbs and nutritional supplements, moreover, alpha-lipoic acid should not be used by pregnant or nursing women, young children, or anyone with liver or kidney disease.

Therapeutic dosages. The most beneficial dosages of alpha-lipoic acid when taken orally have been in the range of 600 to 800 milligrams daily.

Other Supplements with Potential for Nerve-Damage Control

What else in the ever-enlarging world of dietary supplements is showing promise in minimizing nerve damage caused by diabetes? Some preliminary studies of the following supplements have produced encouraging results, but more research needs to be done to establish their effectiveness as well as safety. You should exercise maximum caution by monitoring your blood sugar very carefully if you should decide to try any of these, therefore, and, as always, don't even think about using them without first getting clearance from your doctor.

Acetyl-l-carnitine. This amino acid derivative has been investigated mostly in injected form, but it has produced positive results in several placebo-controlled studies.

Fish oil. Research thus far has been done only with animals but with encouraging results.

Vitamin E and selenium. Preliminary studies have found these two antioxidants to be somewhat helpful in restoring sensation lost to neuropathy, possibly by reducing damage caused by free radicals. (Caution needs to be observed with selenium, however, which can be toxic in dosages exceeding 200 micrograms daily.)

B-complex vitamins (thiamin, pyridoxine, pantethine, cobalamin, inositol). More research needs to be done, but preliminary studies suggest the B vitamins may have some benefit in reducing symptoms of neuropathy in diabetics deficient in these nutrients.

Natural Protection for the Eyes

Diabetes, as you may remember from chapter 1, is the leading cause of blindness in working-age Americans, and it can lead to other vision problems such as cataracts, macular degeneration, and glaucoma as well. Close control of blood sugar levels is the best way to prevent damage to the fragile blood vessels and other highly sensitive tissue of the eyes, but some researchers are optimistic about the protection against eye damage that the following nutrients also may provide.

Vitamin E

Although results have been mixed, some research has found that vitamin E can help increase blood flow to the all-important area of the retina. Some scientists theorize this may help protect this sensitive area by increasing oxygen supplies as well as limiting damage done by free radicals.

Vitamin C

One of vitamin C's roles in the body is to help maintain the strength of connective tissue, the walls of blood vessels, included. This—combined with the discovery that patients with diabetic retinopathy tend to be deficient in vitamin C—has led some scientists to speculate that the nutrient might be helpful in preventing the retinal damage diabetes can cause. Some research suggests vitamin C may help protect against cataracts as well.

Bilberry

Some preliminary studies have shown that powerful antioxidant compounds known as *flavonoids* in this herb may be useful in treating and preventing retinal damage by helping to strengthen

> Vitamin E can help increase blood flow to the all-important area of the retina.

the tiny blood vessels (capillaries) of the eyes. Some test tube studies indicate these flavonoids, like vitamin C, may also be helpful in preventing cataracts.

Natural Protection for the Kidneys and Heart

Of all the organs affected by diabetes, perhaps none gets hit as hard—or with such potential for dire consequences—as the kidneys and heart. While keeping tight control of blood sugar levels is the best way to protect these vital organs, new research is finding that certain natural dietary aids might be able at least to lend a helping hand. Harm to the kidneys and heart is done by more than just high glucose levels, after all: High cholesterol levels, high triglycerides, and elevated levels of sugar-coated (glycosylated) proteins in the blood also can inflict their blows, and it's in areas such as these that some research suggests the following supplements may help.

Stanols

Stanols are cholesterol-lowering substances that occur naturally in plants, now available in modified form in various margarine-type spreads, salad oils, and dietary supplements. They generally can lower total as well as "bad" LDL cholesterol by 10 to 15 percent by inhibiting cholesterol absorption in the intestines, and they have been tested and proven safe in at least 13 double-blind, placebo-controlled studies ranging in length from 1 to 12 months. Because stanols may inhibit the absorption of beta-carotene, however, users are advised to eat plenty of yellow-orange and dark green leafy vegetables such as carrots, kale, spinach, broccoli, and squash to help compensate.

Dietary Fiber

The praises of this supernutrient were sung in chapter 5, but they bear repeating here. Foods high in soluble fiber, especially—such as beans, oats, and most fruits and vegetables—form a gel-like substance in the intestines that can help impede the absorption of cholesterol and glucose alike and hence may help lower not just glucose levels, but risks of heart disease, too.

> *Foods high in soluble fiber form a gel-like substance in the intestines that can help impede the absorption of cholesterol and glucose alike.*

Cold-Water Fish

Fish such as salmon, tuna, mackerel, sardines, haddock, herring, and cod are high in a type of fat known as *omega-3 fatty acids*, which studies show can lower triglyceride levels while also possibly boosting heart-healthy HDLs. Omega-3 fatty acids, in some studies, also have shown an important talent for making red blood cells more "slippery," thus increasing their ability to slip through even the body's tiniest blood vessels to deliver oxygen and other vital nutrients to tissue that might otherwise be short-changed. This may be especially important for people with diabetes, some researchers feel, because the disease by its very nature tends to thicken the blood and impair capillary blood flow.

Vitamin C

Yes, even more kudos for this multitalented nutrient. One double-blind study of 48 people with type 2 diabetes with high cholesterol found that 60 percent of those who took 500 milligrams of vitamin C for a year experienced a 40 percent drop in their total cholesterol levels and a small decrease in their triglyceride levels, too. This study was done more than 20 years ago, and such dramatic results have not been duplicated since, but in light of all vitamin C's other benefits—and its relative safety when taken in reasonable amounts—the nutrient certainly deserves being discussed with your doctor.

Garlic

Studies over the years have produced mixed results with respect to what benefits this pungent bulb may hold for the heart, but taken as a whole, research has produced more positive than negative results. Garlic in some studies has been shown to help lower cholesterol levels, blood pressure, and also the tendency of the blood to clot, all of which can help people with diabetes reduce their elevated risks of heart disease—and flavorfully so.

OTHER TREATMENTS WORTH A TRY

Don't think that complementary medicine stops with herbs and dietary supplements in its efforts to treat diabetes. The "Big D" has the potential to be a very full-body problem, remember, so it offers itself to a variety of alternative healing techniques. As Steven Bratman, M.D., the medical director of TNP.com (The Natural Pharmacist Web site) and author of *The Alternative Medicine Sourcebook* and *The Alternative Medicine Ratings Guide* points out, "Diabetes is such a multifaceted disease that a wide variety of lifestyle changes can affect its treatment—directly, indirectly, and probably a lot of ways in between."

By participating in a support group or art class, for example, people might wind up eating less because they're out of the house for

Lessons in "Quack" Control

As diabetes becomes more prevalent, so, too, do opportunities for quackery. There are enough subtle loopholes in advertising ethics for many totally useless products to squeeze through, the result being the steady flow of quackery we now see in virtually all available media—TV, radio, magazines, newspapers, and now the Internet. How can we know the "worth-a-trys" from the total shams? Common sense should help appreciate the wisdom in these basic tips:

- **Don't fall for star appeal. If a product needs a celebrity to sell it, it's probably because the product doesn't have enough star power of its own.** A case study of one, moreover, is very bad science. Just because a product has allegedly worked for one person doesn't mean it's going to work for others.

- **Don't fall for hyperbole.** Steady progress in treating diabetes is being made, but not in the leaps and bounds some products want to claim. If a product promises results that sound in any way fantastic, consider the product to be just that: a fantasy.

- **Don't fall for a long history—or short one, either.** Some cures hang their hat on being miracle cures "centuries old"—which you should interpret merely as evidence of how ineffective it must be for not being better known. Be just as wary of

those several hours, Dr. Bratman says. In combination with the improvement in mood such activities can foster, and hence better compliance with other aspects of treatment, the therapeutic affect can be very real, indeed. "Alternative therapies often can be a kind of catalyst to better self-care across the board," Dr. Bratman says.

Check out these following spirit sparkers with that in mind. Aside from the obvious physical benefits associated with some of these therapies, the good they can do for your mind may be their greatest bene-

treatments touted to be the "latest." If it really is so recent, then it hasn't had a chance to prove its true worth or safety, either.

- **Do fall for the truth.** If you're looking for the truth, the places to look are organizations in the business of selling fact not fiction—the American Diabetes Association, the American Medical Association, the National Diabetes Education Program, the Joslin Diabetes Center, and the International Diabetes Federation (with more than 100 member nations worldwide). These organizations dedicate themselves to keeping their ears to the ground for the latest developments, evaluate them for efficacy and safety, and then spend billions of dollars to disseminate this information to the public, so these are the outfits to give your attention to when seeking valid claims about the latest treatments for diabetes. But are these bureaucracies too cautious and conservative to be proponents of the most "cutting edge" developments? Only to the point of keeping you from getting "cut." With the emergence of alternative medicine as another major player in the medical marketplace, these organizations have had to become more open than ever to new ideas and new approaches to this age-old problem. You should see them as representing the best of both worlds: the willingness to be new and the dedication to being safe.

fit of all. As always, however, none of these should take the place of conventional medical care, nor should they be tried without the approval and supervision of your primary care doctor.

Relaxation: Learning to Turn Down the Heat

To understand how relaxation may help minimize the dangers of diabetes, it can help to go back a few years—back to our cave-dwelling days when we were more likely to have to deal with a crazed caribou rather than a crazed boss. Those days were more healthful—metabolically speaking—because we either fought or fled, both of which burned up the sudden rush of blood sugar our bodies would produce to give us those options. Now we have few options but to sit and stew when our monstrous managers or 2-hour traffic jams get our blood sugars boiling, the result being greater risks for the high blood pressure, high cholesterol, and other cardiovascular risk factors that tend to haunt people with diabetes even without the added burdens of emotional stress. These individuals, therefore, may have even more to gain by learning to relax than people without the disease.

Not only can learning to relax help control blood pressure and high cholesterol, moreover, studies show it can help control blood sugar, too.

Not only can learning to relax help control blood pressure and high cholesterol, moreover, studies show it can help control blood sugar, too—the fight-or-flight fuel produced by threatening situations in the first place. Many studies have shown that people with diabetes have more trouble controlling their blood sugar when they're also having to control troublesome events in their lives. The good news, though, is that learning to chill out can help bring it all back into line.

We'll be talking more about the mind's role in diabetes in chapter 8, but for now we'll just mention that one recent study found that learning to relax helped some people with the disease lower their glucose levels by between 9 and 12 percent. The director of the study, Angela McGrady, Ph.D., a professor at the Medical College of Ohio in Toledo, offers these basic tips for bringing your anxiety levels down, and possibly your blood sugar levels along with them:

- **Decompress daily.** With our jobs, family responsibilities, and dirty kitchen floors seeming to compete for our every waking moment, it's important to take a "time-out" each day just to let the internal springs unwind, Dr. McGrady says. You can do it by taking 10 or 15 minutes just to sit quietly, lie down, or go for a walk, or you can be more systematic and get professional instruction in a variety of techniques including progressive muscle relaxation, visualization, autogenic training, and meditation. Ask your doctor or member of your health care team for a referral if you think learning to "chill" may be a good idea for you. There are no official licensing agencies for most of these modalities, unfortunately, so word-of-mouth recommendations may be all you'll have to go on.

- **Put a carrot at the end of the stick.** When you know you have a stressful task or event you've got to get through, give yourself something to look forward to after its conclusion— a romantic weekend, a new outfit, a dinner out at a nice restaurant, or a concert or movie. Anything to provide a sense of reward.

- **Don't add fuel to the fire.** Stimulants such as caffeine and nicotine might seem to prime you for battle, but not without leaving your nerves all the more frazzled for the having made the fight.

- **Know when to ask for help.** It's not a sign of weakness but rather wisdom to seek professional help when you're feeling overwhelmed.

SUPPORT GROUPS: "COMRADES IN ADVERSITY"

"Support groups are much more than feel-good get-togethers," write the editors of *Smart Choices in Alternative Medicine*. "Scientific studies have found that support groups can measurably improve participants' health and add years to their lives—even in the case of serious diseases like cancer."

And diabetes. A study done by researchers from Texas Tech University Health Sciences Center found that patients with diabetes

Yoga: Worth the Stretch

Yes, if you'd like to go so far as to stand on your head to help straighten out your blood sugar, you can try that, too—pending your doctor's permission, of course. One study done in India found that 104 of 149 patients with type 2 diabetes were able to reduce their oral medications after taking yoga classes for 40 days, and another found that 40 days of yoga therapy helped 30 patients with type 2 diabetes metabolize glucose more normally when their medications were stopped. Yoga may exert its helpful effects by reducing levels of stress hormones as well as providing some very good exercise, researchers say.

"Yoga postures can be deceiving," says Karrie Demers, M.D., a yoga instructor as well as board-certified internist and medical director of the Center for Health and Healing at the Himalayan Institute in Honesdale, Pennsylvania. "They might appear easy, but many can be very demanding, and especially the longer they're held."

who participated in support groups gained definite advantages in keeping their blood sugar under control. So as much as misery may love company, it seems to like health as well, and company often can be the catalyst to bringing that health to fruit. To find out why, researcher Irving Yolam, M.D., of Stanford University Medical School recently completed an investigation that revealed the following explanations:

- **Knowing you're not alone**. When people realize that others are sharing their same physical as well as emotional struggles, this knowledge in itself can bring relief.

- **Being inspired with hope.** Members of support groups often hear stories of recovery or learning to cope that can be emotionally uplifting.

As proof of that, a study reported in the *Journal of Alternative and Complementary Medicine* found that previously untrained women participating in yoga class for 4 weeks—in addition to gaining both flexibility and strength—boosted their cardiovascular endurance by 21 percent. As a complement to a more conventional aerobic exercise routine, yoga can be especially beneficial, Dr. Demers says.

If you're interested in giving yoga a try, it's best to learn from a qualified instructor. No certification is required to teach yoga, unfortunately, but you should be able to find a good teacher or class by checking with your local hospital, a reputable health club, or your local YMCA or YWCA. As for what style of yoga to pursue—and there are several—you'll probably be most satisfied with hatha yoga, the most popular type and also one that gives a good physical workout while still emphasizing relaxation through proper mind control and breathing.

- **Being inspired with information.** Such reports of recovery and learning to cope also provide information that can be very useful from a practical standpoint.

- **Learning to open up.** By learning to discuss their feelings at meetings, participants feel better but also learn how to relate better to family members, coworkers, and friends.

- **Gaining by giving.** By helping others at meetings, members boost their own spirits and hence do a lot to help themselves.

- **Facing the big picture.** As a group, members often find the courage to wrestle with life's largest issues—such as how unfair life can seem but also the importance of making the best of it that we can.

How to Get Involved

To find a diabetes support group near you, you can check with your doctor or local hospital or library. You also can review your local newspaper's "events" listings, consult your telephone directory, or contact one of these national clearinghouses listed here. Note, too, that if physical limitations make it difficult or impossible for you to leave your home or health care facility, you still can benefit from the group experience by participating in support groups by phone or by computer on the Internet. The national clearinghouses in this list should be able to give you the information you need to get started, or you can try looking up key search words on the Web such as "diabetes self-help groups."

American Self-Help Clearinghouse
St. Claire's Hospital
Denville, New Jersey 07834
Phone: (973) 326-6789
Web site: www.selfhelpgroup.org

National Self-Help Clearinghouse
365 5th Avenue, Suite 3300
New York, NY 10016
Phone: (212) 354-8525
Web site: www.selfhelpweb.org

CHAPTER 8

Diabetes Day-to-Day
Lessons in Taking Charge

❧

D IABETES CAN BE more than just a medical problem, unfortunately. It can be an emotional problem, a sexual problem, a family problem, a work problem, a financial problem—clearly more than just a pain in the pancreas, that's for sure. Perhaps more than any other disease, in fact, diabetes has the potential to disrupt the activities of daily living because it can demand so much, so often, and with such importance. Your blood sugar becomes your life, and it's in your hands every minute of every day, to control or let slip away—perhaps taking your health along with it. It's a tremendous pressure, and it affects not just you but everyone close to you and even some who are not.

But in this seemingly black cloud can be a silver lining, if you know how to look for it, and that's what this chapter is about. It's about learning to deal with the hardships of diabetes in ways that can help you deal with life itself. As you learn to master the self-discipline and positive thinking required to overcome this very demanding disease, you'll be that much better prepared to deal with anything life may throw your way.

Wishful thinking? No, *winning* thinking. As Robert Louis Stevenson learned from his years of coping with tuberculosis, "Life isn't a matter of getting a good hand, but rather of learning how to play a poor hand well." Keep that in mind as you read this chapter. Yes, diabetes is a poor hand, but by no means does it have to be a losing one. It can be a winning one if played right. Many people, on learning they have diabetes, go on to change their lifestyles in ways that leave them healthier than before they had the disease. Health may live in our bodies, after all, but it's born in our minds, nurtured by hard work and hope.

CLEANING YOUR EMOTIONAL HOUSE

To the degree that diabetes strains the body, unfortunately, it also can strain the mind. First there's the emotional shock of being diagnosed, followed immediately by the need to make what can be difficult lifestyle changes. No time to crawl away and heal from the emotional pain. It's got to be "up and at 'em" right away, which can be difficult, to say the least. Not only must you deal with the trauma of learning you have a life-long disease, moreover, you may find yourself having to contend with mood swings caused by the disease itself. High blood sugar levels may make you feel tired and depressed, while low blood sugar can make you feel nervous, anxious, and scared. It's important not to fall into the trap of feeling powerless in the face of these diabetes-induced emotional states. Not only can that be debilitating in itself, it can deter you from understanding and correcting other situations in your life that may, in fact, be the truer sources of negative moods. It's important not to let diabetes become the "fall guy," in other words, for all that may not be going well in your life.

> *Life isn't a matter of getting a good hand, but rather of learning how to play a poor hand well.*
>
> —ROBERT LOUIS STEVENSON

Is there simply no way around the very lousy fact that you have a disease that's never going to go away? The mind is a powerful thing. Coming to grips with the emotional aspects of diabetes can be challenging—as challenging as dealing with the physical demands, in fact—but it can be done, and there are millions of happy and healthy diabetes "veterans" to prove it. Researchers have measured the mood states and quality of life that people with diabetes report as they learn to cope with their conditions over the years, and the findings are very encouraging. Patients who keep their diabetes under good control report that life gets better, not worse. The earliest stages of the disease are the hardest because they require the most adjustment, but after those adjustments are made, patients report that the sailing becomes relatively smooth.

It's important not to fall into the trap of feeling powerless in the face of diabetes-induced emotional states.

Might this period of adjustment be shortened, thus saving heartache as well as health? Shortened yes, but avoided altogether, probably not—nor should it be. As Wendy Satin Rapaport, L.C.S.W., Psy.D., explains in her excellent book, *When Diabetes Hits Home*, a period of grieving is necessary with diabetes just as with any tragic life event. Negative emotions have to be purged before more positive ones can take their place. "If you do not fulfill your need to complete the grieving process, you risk being continually depressed, anxious, nonadherent, or in denial," Dr. Rapaport says.

It's important to get your period of emotional turmoil out of your system, in other words, so you can build your treatment on a foundation that's emotionally stable. This tumultuous period is likely to consist not just of sadness, moreover, but also anger for being saddled with such a fate, fear of long-term consequences, denial in the hope it all might just go away, and even guilt for feeling partially responsible for your plight. Whatever the gamut of emotions you wind up experiencing, however, it's important that you arrive at one particular emotion at the end, Dr. Rapaport says—acceptance. Not until you've accepted your condition, after all, can you begin to master it.

WHAT IT TAKES TO WIN

What mental skills might mastering diabetes require? In researching that important question, certain key concepts keep emerging. According to experts representing the American Diabetes Association, the International Diabetes Center, and the Harvard Medical School's Joslin Diabetes Center in Boston, the coping strategies that seem to help people deal with diabetes best are those described in the following sections.

Be Determined

There's no way around this one, unfortunately, because controlling diabetes takes work. It takes regular glucose monitoring, paying attention to diet, getting enough exercise, and using medication properly, whether it be insulin, oral medication, or some combination of the two. It also may require periodic checkups for potential complications or possibly even therapy sessions if any such complications have already begun. These are not impossible sacrifices to make, however, especially considering the payoffs, so the

> *Considering the payoffs, the sooner you can accept the basic workload of diabetes, the better.*

sooner you can accept the basic workload of diabetes, the better. And if you need motivation, just remind yourself of the results of the Diabetes Control and Complications Trial mentioned earlier in this book, which found that keeping glucose levels under good control can reduce the risks of some of the potentially most serious complications of diabetes—damage to the nerves and eyes, for example—by as much as 70 percent.

Be Flexible

This might seem like a contradiction to being determined, but it's not. Even with the most diligent attempts at glucose control, unexplainable fluctuations will occur, and it's far better to accept them than to be upset by them. You do yourself an emotional disservice to become upset, but you also put yourself at a physical disadvantage because emotional stress can make blood sugar levels even harder to control, causing it to rise in some people and fall in others. Staying on as even an emotional keel as possible is the best way around this problem, and this applies not just to inexplicable glucose fluctuations but to treatment disruptions in general. If you're forced to miss an exercise session, for example, or you can't get precisely the food you want at a restaurant, don't add insult to injury by letting it upset you. Roll with it, and simply get back on schedule when you can.

Be Honest with Yourself

Sorry, but it will do no good to try to candy-coat your condition if you in fact think it's a royal pain. Such denial could take some of the zeal out of your commitment to overcome your diabetes, and it could prevent you from being as truthful as you should be with your doctor about how you're really feeling. Some patients make the mistake of denying the seriousness of their condition for years, and frequently they suffer serious consequences as a result. Don't make that mistake. The sooner you can declare all-out war against your diabetes, the better. And don't be afraid to let family and friends in on the fervor of your campaign. As we'll see, they can be valuable allies in your treatment efforts.

Be Honest with Others

This may entail risks—such as being nagged about sticking to treatment, or being felt sorry for, or even being shown unfair treatment at work (discussed later), but these risks are outweighed by what stands to be gained. By being truthful with family and friends about your condition, you can be assured they'll be there for you—emotionally as well as physically—in your times of greatest need.

By being honest, you also avoid the highly inadvisable situation of having to hide your condition in ways that could seriously compromise your treatment. You could feel compelled to make unwise dietary decisions at social events, for example, or avoid testing your glucose when you know you should, or even miss an insulin injection simply to avoid being found out. It's not worth it. Let the world around you know about your little "secret," and you won't have to go through the stress—not to mention medical dangers—of having to keep it a secret at all. You also will have that many more shoulders to lean on in times of need.

Don't Be Lulled by the Good Times

Diabetes can be an especially challenging disease to control because it doesn't always seem to need to be controlled. Unlike having a cold, when you might be reminded to take an antihistamine by a stuffy nose, diabetes rarely shows such obvious signs. You might consider it a paradox, in fact, that the better you *do* manage your diabetes, the less it will let you know that it needs to be managed at all. You'll be feeling fine, your blood sugar levels will be within an acceptable range, so your tendency might be to relax your efforts. Don't fall into this trap. Yes, the "lion" may be sleeping, but only because you're doing what's necessary to keep it that way. Try to remember this when things are going well, and just keep doing what you're doing. If you can stay vigilant during such times of peace, you may never have to experience the ravages of war at all.

> *By being truthful with family and friends about your condition, you can be assured they'll be there for you—emotionally as well as physically—in your times of greatest need.*

Keep Your Sense of Humor

This tip comes last, but it just as easily could have appeared first. Research shows that our bodies seem to like a good laugh as much as we do. Laboratory studies have found that people experience a boost in the germ-fighting power of their immune systems when shown funny movies, and other research has shown humor to be a potent remedy for stress.

But what could possibly be funny about diabetes? Nothing, which is why humor can be so useful in helping us deal with it. "Humor can serve as a social lubricant that can help us face rather than deny the seriousness of diabetes," Dr. Rapaport says. Properly used, therefore, humor does not belittle the seriousness of diabetes but rather acknowledges it, allowing us to communicate about circumstances that otherwise might be too difficult. As it can do with all potentially grave situations, moreover, humor can serve as a valuable defuser of stress while also fostering the kind of positive mind-set important for keeping us energized in our treatment efforts. As Mark Gorkin, a therapist and stand-up comedian recommends, we should "let the farce be with us."

DIABETES AND SEX

Can diabetes affect sexual function? Unfortunately, yes. In men and women alike, diabetes that's not well controlled can begin to damage blood vessels and nerves responsible for the blood flow and sensation that play an important role in sexual performance. In men this performance failure generally takes the form of erectile dysfunction—the inability to obtain or sustain an erection sufficient for intercourse—while in women the problem is usually a decrease in vaginal lubrication and loss of feeling in the vaginal area. Women also may develop other symptoms that can cause sexual interference, such as menstrual irregularity, yeast infections of the vaginal area, urinary tract infections (also a problem for men), and loss of bladder control. If you're a woman suffering from any of these complications, consult with your doctor. Infections can be treated with antibiotics, and vaginal dryness often can be helped with a lubricant.

> *Humor does not belittle the seriousness of diabetes but rather acknowledges it, allowing us to communicate about circumstances that otherwise might be too difficult.*

Sexual function also can sometimes be refurbished with estrogen taken orally or administered to the vaginal area directly in the form of a suppository.

The important thing to remember—whether you're a man or women—is that complications do not have to mean your days of sexual pleasure are behind you. There are therapies that can help. Remember, too, that better sex and better blood sugar control tend to go hand in hand, so the better you take care of your diabetes, the better you'll be taking care of your sex life. Use that as incentive if it helps. Also keep in mind, however, that good sex can be like good exercise: It burns calories and hence glucose, so you may need to make medication adjustments or have a snack before or after a soiree to keep low blood sugar at bay.

> *The better you take care of your diabetes, the better you'll be taking care of your sex life.*

Impotence: A Closer Look

If you're a man suffering from sexual dysfunction, you'll first need to determine whether your diabetes is in fact the cause. In the general male population, impotence is caused more often by psychological than physical factors; tests can determine whether this is true in your case. Generally speaking, however, psychological impotence usually comes on suddenly, while impotence for physical reasons tends to develop more slowly, so this in itself can serve as a clue. Even if your impotence is physical in origin, however, its cause could be something other than your diabetes. Trauma to the penis can cause erectile failure, as can other factors such as certain medications used for high blood pressure and depression, shortages of the male hormone testosterone, certain forms of cardiovascular disease, indiscriminate use of alcohol, and smoking. It's important to see your doctor to have these possibilities ruled out before you go saddling your diabetes with the blame.

And if your diabetes is the cause? Fortunately, modern science has fully realized the importance of intercourse as a human function, as exemplified by the novel ways that have been devised to preserve sexual performance despite considerable odds. For men who still have the will, science has found them a way. This is because as serious as diabetes can become, it rarely robs a man of his ability to achieve orgasm. Erections can be difficult to achieve or maintain, but the nerves and other mechanisms responsible for ejaculation in most cases remain intact, leaving just the means to achieving this end to be restored. The following sections describe impotence treatments currently available that have had encouraging success.

> *A s serious as diabetes can become, it rarely robs a man of his ability to achieve orgasm.*

Viagra

Taken approximately an hour before sex, the all-too-publicized drug sildenafil (Viagra) has been shown to work in 70 percent of men with diabetes, although side effects may include headaches, facial flushing, indigestion, and blurred or slightly colored vision. It shouldn't be used more than once a day, however, nor should it be used in conjunction with nitrate drugs such as nitroglycerine used to treat chest pains caused by heart disease, because possibly fatal drops in blood pressure could occur.

Penile Injections

Self-administered about 30 minutes prior to sex, these injections use one of several drugs (papaverine, phentolamine, or most recently alprostadil) that increase blood flow to the penis by causing blood vessels within the organ to dilate. They've been found to be effective in 85 to 95 percent of men with diabetes, and although side effects are minimal, they can include pain, bruising, the formation of nodules at the injection site, and, in certain rare cases, a potentially serious condition known as *priapism* in which the penis remains erect long after its mission has been accomplished. If the condition persists for longer than 4 hours, an injection to "deflate" the penis is required.

Penile Suppositories

As the name indicates, this method employs a tubular device that, when inserted into the opening at the tip of the penis and then squeezed, delivers a small pill containing alpoprostadil, the same vasodilator used via injection mentioned earlier. Advantages of this method include the option of varying the dosage and hence potency of medication delivered and also frequency: While injections should not be used more than once in 24 hours or more than three times in any given week, "MUSE," as the suppository system is called, permits usage twice within a 24-hour period.

Vacuum Devices

This method sucks blood into the penis by way of a pump attached to a tube that fits over the organ like a sleeve. Once enough blood has been summoned to produce a satisfactory erection, a rubber band is placed around the base of the penis to keep the blood from escaping. While the method is capable of sustaining rigidity for up to 30 minutes, it can produce pain and numbness, and it has the additional drawback of sometimes choking off the flow of semen, thus preventing ejaculation.

Penile Implants

For the truly committed, this system is available in a permanently semirigid form or as an inflatable version that is made rigid by a manually operated pump, housed along with the testicles inside the scrotal sac, which readies the implant for use by filling it with fluid when squeezed. Either way, surgery is required to imbed the necessary hardware, and although difficult for some men to fathom, the system has been used safely and effectively by many.

DIABETES AND THE WORKPLACE

How much should you let your coworkers or employer know about your diabetes? If you'd feel more comfortable not having your illness known, that's your call to make, but it will require the effort and stress of keeping your condition a secret, which could risk compromising your treatment. Many experts feel more is to be gained than lost by letting diabetes be known at the workplace, especially as a safety precaution should you suffer from an acute attack of high or low blood sugar, because you can educate your coworkers on how to help. Besides, laws are now in place that are designed to protect you against unfair treatment because of your disease. One is called the Americans with Disabilities Act of 1990, and the U.S. Court of Appeals was obliged to rule in 1998 that it had to include people with diabetes working for companies consisting of at least 15 employees. The law states:

> The determination that an individual poses a "direct threat" shall
> be based on an individualized assessment of the individual's present
> ability to safely perform the essential functions of the job.

What this means is that someone with diabetes can't be discriminated against with respect to being hired, fired, promoted, trained, or paid as long as they are capable of doing their job effectively and safely. Nor can someone be asked by an employer whether he or she has diabetes. Someone with diabetes *can* be asked to pass a physical examination to prove capability of performing a certain job, however, but rarely is this a problem for people who keep their diabetes under good control.

L aws are now in place that are designed to protect you against unfair treatment because of your disease.

Another law to be aware of is the Family and Medical Leave Act, passed in 1993, which allows employees of companies of 50 people or more to take as many as 12 weeks off each year, unpaid, to care for their own illness or to take care of a family member who is seriously ill. The time may be taken in a single 12-week stretch or in shorter periods such as one day a week, and the employee must continue to be covered under the company's health insurance policy. Usually a

30-day notice must be given, however, and the employee must have accumulated at least a year (or 1,250 hours) of service to qualify.

What do you do if your company refuses to comply with either of these laws? If it happens, you do have recourse. If you encounter a situation in which you feel you're being unfairly treated by your employer because of your diabetes, contact one or more of the following agencies until you get things straightened out. You might need the help of a lawyer if the going gets tough, but it can be worth the effort. Good luck.

- The Equal Employment Opportunity Commission, 1801 L Street N.W., Washington, D.C., 10507; call (800) 669-4000 to find your local affiliate.

- The Disability Rights Education and Defense Fund, Inc., 2212 6th Street, Berkeley, CA 94710; (510) 644-2555.

- Your state or local Department of Labor or Employment.

- Your union representative. If you belong to a union, its Employment Discrimination Office may be able to help.

- Your state or local bar association. They may be able to help you find a legal representative willing to take your case pro bono, which means with no cost.

- The U.S. Department of Justice Disability Rights Section, P.O. Box 66738, Washington, D.C., 20035; (800) 514-0301.

DIABETES AND MEDICAL INSURANCE

There's good news and bad news regarding getting medical insurance if you have diabetes. The good news is that yes, you can get it; but the bad news is that you may have to shop around, and it could cost you more. Generally you're better off approaching large group insurers that will be better able to spread greater costs around should those costs occur. Whomever you approach, however, here are some key issues to get straight before you sign on any dotted lines:

- What is the total annual cost, and how often will payment be required?

- Is there a deductible, and if so, how much?

- Is there a copayment fee, which means part of every cost you incur will be your responsibility to pay?

- Will the plan pay for durable medical equipment such as an insulin pump should you need it at some point after you enroll?

- To what extent will the program pay for medications and supplies, and is there a restriction on what types?

- Will you be covered for treatment by specialists such as ophthalmologists and podiatrists?

- Does the policy dictate what physicians, hospitals, or labs you may use?

- Is home health care included under the policy, and to what extent?

Note: Often you may need to be persistent to be reimbursed for certain services, but keep at it. Some insurers can even be persuaded to foot the bill for services or equipment not originally specified in your policy if you and your health care team present a concerted and united front.

TIPS FOR TAKING YOUR DIABETES ON VACATION

It's important to continue to live life to the fullest when diabetes strikes, the experts agree, so if you enjoy traveling, don't think your diabetes has to stop you. You just need to be well packed and well prepared, which the following tips can help you do:

- **Have a medical checkup.** In addition to giving you the confidence that your diabetes is well enough under control to travel, a checkup can give you an opportunity to have your doctor

write a letter explaining the details of your condition should it
be needed in case of an emergency. The letter could come in
handy, too, should you be questioned about the purpose of
your suspicious-looking collection of medications, syringes,
and vials.

- **Immunize early.** If you're traveling to where immunizations
are required, try to get them at least a month before your de-
parture to allow your doctor time to check for any adverse reactions on your glucose control.

- **Travel heavy.** Whatever medications or supplies are involved
in your blood sugar control, take twice as much as you think
you'll need, just to play it safe. Also have your doctor write pre-
scriptions for all the medications you take so that you can get
more should your supplies be stolen or lost.

- **Don't be duped by time zones**. If your trip is taking you
across several time zones, check with your doctor on whether
you'll need to adjust your insulin or medication schedule accordingly.

- **Stay active on long trips.** Whether it's a long plane, train, bus,
or car ride, try not to let more than about an hour and a half go
by without at least getting up to walk or stretch to promote circulation to the extremities. You'll feel better and reduce risks of
blood clots, too.

- **Identify yourself.** This means carrying a card in your wallet as
well as a name tag on your wrist or neck that explains your condition, the medication you take, and the name and number of a
doctor to call in case of an emergency. (You can get such a
number by having your doctor locate a physician where you'll
be visiting ahead of time or by contacting the International
Diabetes Federation once you arrive.)

- **Learn the language**. In case of an emergency, it can be helpful to
be able to say, "Please give me some fruit juice or something to

eat," or, "How can I find a doctor?" in the local language. To play it doubly safe, carry a piece of paper bearing these same messages should a severe bout of blood sugar leave you speechless.

- **Don't go hungry.** Traveling frequently takes you out of control of when meals are served, so try to keep snacks with you to avoid having to go long periods without eating. This becomes especially important on long car trips that require your full competency at the wheel.

- **Be careful when sampling strange foods.** The filet of water buffalo might be a chance of a lifetime, so go for it, but do at least monitor your glucose levels often when eating unusual foods for the first time. You may learn that it should be the last.

- **Be extra vigilant against digestive distress.** We're talking about diarrhea here, and also motion sickness, both of which can cause major disruptions in the all-important balance between blood sugar and medication levels—insulin, especially. Diarrhea can best be avoided by drinking bottled water only or tea made from boiled water and by being wary of undercooked meats and milk products, including cream sauces and cheese. To avoid motion sickness, ask your health care team to recommend an effective medication.

- **Prevent sunburn.** The stress to the skin caused by excessive sun exposure can raise blood sugar levels dramatically, so wear a high-numbered sunblock if you can't avoid the sun altogether, supplemented possibly by a wide-brimmed hat and long sleeves. Consider a suntan, in other words, one souvenir you can do without.

A WORD ON DRUGS

We're referring to the illegal ones this time, and we need to because people with diabetes are prey to the same pressures and temptations as anyone in today's tumultuous world. People with diabetes may even be more vulnerable to illegal drugs because of the physical as well as emotional hardships they must endure. Is there a place for drugs in providing escape from these strains? Not considering the price. In addition to entailing the risk called jail, illegal drugs can impair the judgment needed for consistent adherence to treatment while also directly causing harmful swings in blood sugar. Marijuana, for example, can drive glucose levels down, but then back up as the "munchies" take hold. Cocaine, heroine, and amphetamines, on the other hand, can drive blood sugar up while negating the good sense needed to do something about it. Drugs and diabetes, therefore, should be seen as a risky mix even without the long list of other health hazards drugs are known to entail. The diabetic body is challenged enough as it is without having to endure the assaults on the cardiovascular, respiratory, and immune systems that drugs can mount.

> *Illegal drugs can impair the judgment needed for consistent adherence to treatment while also directly causing harmful swings in blood sugar.*

THE CHILD WITH DIABETES

The greatest challenge of all associated with diabetes may be raising a child with the disease. The child's care can invade every aspect of family life, thus making the disease, in a sense, the entire family's disease. The going may get especially tough during adolescence as children begin to test the authoritative waters, and aspects of treatment become power struggles or just another rule to break. It's these times especially that can test your commitment, patience, and love. The good news, though, is that children have the potential to be the most compliant patients of all because they haven't had decades to become set in their ways—hence the importance of getting them off to a good start.

We have space here, unfortunately, to give you only a brief outline of strategies to employ and goals to shoot for. And notice we said "shoot for." It's tough enough to keep oneself on a tight treatment schedule much less a teenager or toddler, so don't expect perfection. Do expect to communicate as honestly and lovingly as you can, however, that yes, diabetes may be "unfair" but that resisting treatment is only going to make it more of an injustice by allowing it to run its cruel course.

Note: As explained in chapter 1, most children diagnosed with diabetes are found to have type 1, which requires injections of insulin because the body has lost all ability to make its own. Type 2, however, in which the body produces insulin only to have it rejected by the body's cells, is becoming increasingly common among children as obesity and lack of exercise also have been on the rise.

> *Children have the potential to be the most compliant patients of all because they haven't had decades to become set in their ways.*

- **Deal with the present**. When your child is diagnosed with diabetes, don't waste emotional energy worrying about long-term complications. Your first concerns should be to learn the basics of day-to-day care, thus not wasting any time in keeping future problems at bay.

- **Know what you'll need to know.** You might feel overwhelmed at first as you hear of what your child's treatment may require, but it should be less daunting if you can segment the seeming morass of information into the following seven categories. Once these basic aspects of treatment are straight in your mind, it should be easier as you sit down with your child's doctor to learn the details of each:

  1. How to give an insulin injection.
  2. How to recognize and treat symptoms of low blood sugar.
  3. How to recognize and treat symptoms of high blood sugar.
  4. How to test your child's blood sugar and urine (for ketones).
  5. The best foods for your child to eat, and on what schedule.

6. How exercise will affect your child's dietary and medication needs.

7. How to make adjustments when your child becomes ill.

- **Don't be *too* demanding about diet.** While it can be tempting to want to control your child's every bite, you should know that the nutritional needs of children are no different from those of children without the disease. If anything, it's better for a growing child's blood sugar to run slightly on the high rather than low side to assure that adequate glucose is available for proper development. This is by no means free license for your child to pig out on junk food, but it is to suggest that more may be gained than lost by a modest amount of leniency, and certainly if the struggle is going to cause alienation.

- **Don't go it alone.** While it's true that the bulk of the responsibility of caring for your child's diabetes will lie with you as the child's parent, it's important to share the load—with other family members, with relatives, with caretakers you trust, and with qualified personnel at your child's school. You need to feel confident that your child is in good hands other than just your own. Also consider it critical to stay in close communication with your child's health care team concerning any questions or problems that may arise. It can be helpful, too, to join a support group consisting of other caretakers in your position to share victories as well as defeats. Check with the American Diabetes Association or the Juvenile Diabetes Association on how to find a group near you.

- **Try to be sympathetic to the special concerns of teenagers.** Adolescence can be an especially difficult time for children to comply with the treatment demands of diabetes because it tends to be a time of rebellion against authority in general. Treatment involves rules, and *rule* for many children at this age is the worst of the four-letter words. Then, too, this is a time when children may be tempted to forego treatment guidelines to see whether they really in fact have a serious disease. Teenage girls, moreover, may be motivated to skimp on insulin injections given the societal pressure they feel to control their weight. This is not to imply that such behaviors should be condoned but rather only understood so that you might more intelligently argue against them.

- **Stay as positive as possible.** Yes, caring for your child with diabetes will at times be exhausting and even exasperating, but you do everyone a big favor by trying to stay as upbeat as possible. Your attitude of hope—or hopelessness—will certainly be picked up by your child, so it will be important to set the most positive example you can. In addition to keeping your chin up despite the daily demands of this disease, this will mean doing your best to avoid quarrels that may arise over treatment issues, especially ones arising from any sort of blame associated with your child's illness. It's no one's "fault"—genetically or in any other way—so try to come together as a team that's going to win no matter what.

- **Don't forget the well ones.** It's not uncommon for the siblings of a diabetic child to feel neglected as they see so much attention pass them by. Not only can this be bad for them; it can be bad for their sick brother or sister who usually will suffer in some way from the resentment. Being careful to ration your attention somewhat evenly can help prevent this unhealthy dynamic.

- **Read a good book.** To learn more about parenting a child with diabetes, you can consult many good books, some of which are listed here. Those marked with asterisks are written to be understood by children, too.

The Best Year of My Life, Book One: Getting Diabetes by Jed Block (Jed Block, 1999)*

Diabetes in Children: A Guide for the Family by Arlan L. Rosenbloom (Health Information Network, 1996)

Growing Up With Diabetes: What Children Want Their Parents To Know by Alicia McAuliffe (John Wiley & Sons, 1998)

My Own Type 1 Diabetes Book by Sandra J. Hollenberg (Grandma Sandy, 2000)*

The Sun, the Rain and the Insulin: Growing Up with Diabetes by Joan McCracken (Tiffen Press, 1996)*

Sweet Kids: How to Balance Diabetes Control and Good Nutrition with Family Peace by Betty Page Brackenridge (American Diabetes Association, 1996)

Taking Diabetes to School by Kim Gosselin (JayJo Books, 1998)*

The Ten Keys to Helping Young Children Grow Up With Diabetes: A Practical Guide for Parents & Caregivers by Tim Wysocki (American Diabetes Association, 1997)

A Word on "Word Rage": Think Before You Hurt

It can be easy to say some pretty hurtful things in the arguments that can occur with children over treatment issues, but it's important not to because of the lasting emotional damage it can do. Words said in a moment can cause pain for a lifetime, and it's just not worth the momentary sense of release. As Wendy Satin Rapaport says in *When Diabetes Hits Home,* we shouldn't speak when our hearts are full of anger, just as we should not speak when our mouths are full of food. Try giving yourself 10 minutes to "digest" your angry feelings before spitting them out. You can save yourself a lot of emotional cleanup in the years ahead if you do.

Juvenile Diabetes: The Signs to Look For

What signs should alert you that a child of yours could have diabetes? If the child is old enough to speak, he or she may complain of fatigue, blurred vision, difficulty breathing, or pain in the stomach or legs. Other common signs to look for—which can be helpful in indicating diabetes in children too young to speak—include frequent urination or bed-wetting, unusual thirst, irritability, and weight loss despite a good appetite. It's important to know, too, that unlike the slow-developing symptoms of type 2 diabetes, which is the type more common in adults, symptoms of type 1 diabetes—the type more common in children—are likely to appear suddenly and progress very rapidly. It's important not to take a wait-and-see attitude, therefore, if a child begins to show any suspicious signs. Usually a simple blood test by your child's pediatrician is all that's required for diabetes to be diagnosed.

WHEN TO GET HELP

Even the best coping strategies and strongest of wills can get mired in the emotional muck diabetes can put in our paths, and it's important to get help when this occurs. A positive frame of mind is just too important in dealing with diabetes to allow yourself to feel depressed. Depression can influence blood sugar levels directly by affecting hormone levels but also indirectly by affecting adherence to treatment, so it's definitely not something to assume is just going to go away or is simply "par" for the diabetes course. If you've been experiencing two or more of the following symptoms on a daily basis for more than 2 weeks, a talk with your doctor or other member of your health care team is definitely in order:

☐   You've been having trouble sleeping.

☐   You have little or no appetite.

☐   You feel tired all the time.

☐   You've been having trouble thinking clearly.

☐   Nothing seems to interest you anymore.

☐   Nothing seems funny to you anymore.

☐   You feel worthless.

☐   You often think of suicide.

It's possible that your depressed moods are simply a result of poor blood sugar control, but if not, your doctor can advise you on the next best step to take. If it's advised to see a therapist, you're likely to be amazed at the amount of good a little "talk therapy" can do. Counselors who specialize in diabetes often can provide subtle but key perspectives that help patients see even the seemingly most hopeless situations in a very different light. Besides, depression by its very nature shuts the mind down to the very sort of positive and problem-solving thinking that hard times require. Many medications are now available that also can give positive thinking a boost, so you should remain open to this option as well.

Last but not least, studies show that support groups (see chapter 7) can do a world of good in helping people with diabetes through their most troubled times, as can counseling from a trusted representative of your religious faith, so check on these options, too. The bottom line is that staying on top of diabetes is going to require all of you—mind, body, and soul.

CHAPTER 9

On the Horizon
An End in Sight

W HAT MIGHT THE future hold for this disease that's been ravaging humankind since it was described by the ancient Egyptians as causing the body to "melt" away back in 1500 B.C.?

Pose that question to the person who keeps watch over the Juvenile Diabetes Research Foundation International (JDRFI)—the leading funder of diabetes research in the world—and you better have some time on your hands. "There's so much going on right now, and all of it so encouraging that it's hard to know where to begin," says Marc Hurlbert, Ph.D., the scientific program manager of the JDRFI. "New scientific technologies are allowing us to make break-through discoveries that might have been unthinkable even just a few years ago."

Combine this with the incredible communication that now exists between the various scientific fields studying this disease and you've got knowledge accelerating in an exponential fashion, Dr. Hurlbert says. "We've probably made more progress toward finding a cure for diabetes in the past 5 or 6 years than in the previous 3,500 years," he says.

Diabetes, in other words, is a disease on its deathbed. Some key pieces of the puzzle still need to be put into place before scientists confidently will be able to give us a timeline on a cure, but at the rate things are going, it's "inevitable" that one will be found, Dr. Hurlbert says. Until that illusive cure is achieved, however, you may certainly expect many important advances in other key areas of diabetes treatment, including more effective medications, pain-free glucose monitoring techniques, improved diagnostic procedures, and better ways of predicting who'll develop the disease in the first place.

BETTER GLUCOSE MONITORING: MORE ACCURACY, LESS "OUCH"

For many people with diabetes, glucose control wouldn't be such a problem if glucose monitoring weren't such a problem. To go poking one's fingers with a lancet to draw blood several times a day is painful in addition to just being a pain. Sensitive to this, scientists have been hard at work to devise simpler and more comfortable monitoring procedures, some of which are available now. Others should be available soon, needing only to receive final approval from the federal Food and Drug Administration (FDA). Here's a look at some of the more promising of these products, designed to make "ouch" obsolete.

Sampling by Suction

Called the Vaculance Lancing Device, this unit can be set to draw blood from four different depths, which it does by creating a vacuum once the skin has been lightly punctured. This causes less pain than conventional pricking devices and also offers the advantage of allowing blood to be drawn from areas of the body such as the arms, legs, and abdomen, thus eliminating the "fingers as pincushion" syndrome. The Vaculance Lancing Device is made by the Bayer Corporation, must be used with disposable test strips, and costs about $40.

Lancing with a Laser

"Beam me up that blood sample, Scotty." Glucose monitoring can be almost that simple with the Lasette, which uses a minutely focused beam of light to burn a tiny hole in the skin rather than puncturing it mechanically. Some discomfort is involved, but much less than with a lancing device, its manufacturer says. The Lasette uses a cartridge good for 120 tests that costs $15, and it is highly portable at a weight of only 9 ounces. It is not light on the pocketbook, however, with the personal model costing about $1,000 and the professional model twice that much. The Lasette is made by Cell Robotics International.

Extraction by Electricity

Called the GlucoWatch Biographer, this clever gadget uses electrical current to draw glucose painlessly into a patch worn on the inside of a device that looks like a wristwatch, which then gives readings every 20 to 30 minutes. A recent study reported in the *Journal of the American Medical Association* found the system to be more accurate at assessing glucose levels than even two pin pricks every hour. Available already in Europe, the device still is awaiting final FDA approval in the United States, unfortunately, but should be available sometime this year for about $250.

The GlucoWatch Biographer uses electrical current to draw glucose painlessly into a patch worn on the inside of a device that looks like a wristwatch.

Another company exploring the "patch" approach to measuring blood glucose is Technical Chemicals and Products Inc., whose patch is worn on the forearm. After about 5 minutes, the patch is assessed with a small electronic meter. This handy system still is undergoing clinical trials.

"Test Me Under My Skin"

That wish can be granted by a "continuous glucose monitoring system" known as the MiniMed, manufactured by MiniMed Technologies, which consists of a tiny sensing device implanted beneath the skin of the abdomen. The sensor then gives readings every 5 minutes of the amount of glucose, not in the blood but rather in the interstitial fluid (ISF) that surrounds the body's cells. This information is then downloaded into a computer in your physician's office such that a very accurate profile of glucose levels extending over a 72-hour period can be attained. The system, which has been approved by the FDA for physician but not patient use, is intended to supplement conventional glucose monitoring, not replace it. Studies have shown it can be of significant benefit in helping physicians work with their patients to keep glucose levels under control. Ask your physician to look into the MiniMed system if you're interested. In the future, plans are to coordinate the MiniMed system with another implanted device capable of delivering insulin in direct response to the glucose readings received.

Skin Unscathed

Perhaps the most ingenious of all is the apparatus that requires nothing to be extracted from the skin at all. Called the Diasensor 1000, made by Biocontrol Technology Inc., it looks a bit like a desktop copying machine and uses a fiber-optic pulse of infrared light to measure glucose levels as a patient merely lays his or her forearm on top of the device. Like the GlucoWatch Biographer, the Diasensor is already being sold in Europe but is still awaiting the official go-ahead from the FDA in the United States. At an anticipated $9,000, the Diasensor will not be cheap, however. Its manufacturers point out that it requires no disposable supplies of any kind, however, which is noteworthy given that test strips alone for most conventional glucose monitoring systems can cost many patients as much as $150 a month.

> *The Diasensor 1000 uses a fiber-optic pulse of infrared light to measure glucose levels as a patient merely lays his or her forearm on top of the device.*

Long-Term Testing Also on the Way

Yes, even tests for hemoglobin A1c—the substance that indicates long-term blood sugar levels—will be available soon. Developed by Metrika, Inc., the DRx HbA1c Patient Monitor reveals in just 8 minutes average glucose levels over the preceding 90 days. Approved already by the FDA for use by physicians, it should be available for use by patients by the time this book goes to print.

NEEDLE-FREE INSULIN

Medications have been the mainstay of diabetes treatment since the discovery of insulin more than 80 years ago, and this will continue as science proceeds to fine-tune its pharmaceutical assault. Drugs for controlling blood sugar will continue to be improved and made safer with fewer side effects, and more medications for combating complications of diabetes will become available. Even drugs for assisting weight loss now are entering the medication arsenal.

Perhaps the most eagerly awaited progress, however, has been in the area of needle-free systems for delivering insulin. Several approaches have met with great success in clinical trials and were on the brink of FDA approval as this book was going to print. Here's a quick rundown of the methods scientists have been working on—some of which could be available by the time you read this. Check with your doctor to be sure.

Insulin via Inhalation

Scientists have been searching for a way to deliver insulin to the bloodstream without having to inject it ever since the lifesaving hormone was discovered back in the early 1920s, but their efforts have been stymied by several problems. Insulin taken by mouth is destroyed by the process of digestion, and to get insulin into the bloodstream by way of the nose has been hampered by poor transport of insulin through the mucous membranes of the nasal passages. These routes of administration are still being explored, as we'll be seeing in a moment, but what has met with the most encouraging success has been inhaling a powdered form of insulin into the lungs directly by way of the mouth. This puts insulin in contact with the highly permeable tissue of the lungs.

Researchers have had such success with this method that an insulin inhaler has entered the final stages of FDA approval and should be available by the summer or fall of 2002. Made by Inhale Therapeutic Systems, Inc., working with Pfizer, Inc., the device is a portable unit about the size of a flashlight that works similarly to the type of inhalers used by people with asthma. The device is loaded with measured doses of insulin in powdered form, a trigger is pulled to disperse the insulin as a cloud into a chamber at the top of the inhaler, and with one slow, deep breath, delivery is completed. The method bypasses the problem of colds and upper respiratory infections, although researchers concede it may produce variable results in people who have asthma or chronic obstructive lung disease, such as emphysema, or who smoke.

How well has it worked? In studies done with people with type 1 and type 2 diabetes, use of the inhaler was found to control blood sugar levels as well as injected insulin, and with such convenience that 80 percent of the type 1 patients and 92 percent of the type 2 patients chose to continue using the device at the conclusion of the 3-month trials. What's more, scientists are hopeful that inhaled insulin might have potential for preventing type 1 diabetes in children, a hope based on research showing that the disease sometimes can be avoided if children are treated with insulin early enough to keep the disease from doing pancreatic damage.

Oral Insulin

In addition to inhaled insulin, scientists have been working on ways to administer insulin orally, and here, too, great progress is being made. Perhaps the most promising product based on the results of studies done so far has been a liquid formulation called Oralin, administered in the form of a spray similar to a nasal decongestant that enters the bloodstream through the skin on the inside of the cheeks. Made by the Generex Biotechnology Corporation, Oralin has been performing well in studies of type 1 and 2 patients conducted at the Diabetes and Glandular Disease Clinic in San Antonio, Texas, and should be available within a few years. "The results of these trials have been very positive, and signify a significant breakthrough in alternative insulin delivery," said Oralin research director Sherwyn Schwartz, M.D., in response to results of the product's latest series of tests.

One liquid formulation, called Oralin, is administered in the form of a spray that enters the bloodstream through the skin on the inside of the cheeks.

Other methods to administer insulin orally that currently are being explored include a patch that would provide insulin in a time-released fashion when placed inside the mouth (being investigated by Noven Pharmaceuticals) and also the long-sought-after insulin pill. Cortecs International of London, for example, is exploring a method of coating insulin in an enzyme-resistant resin that helps carry the fragile hormone through the digestive system unharmed. The method thus far has worked well enough in pigs, Cortecs reports, that human trials will be the next step. Other efforts to create a diabetes pill include those by researchers at Brown University who've had success in encasing insulin in plastic beads that don't dissolve until they reach the bloodstream. And scientists from the University of Maryland have been working at facilitating the passage of insulin into the bloodstream by using a substance (produced by the microbe responsible for cholera) that their studies show makes the walls of the small intestine more permeable.

Taken as a whole, the efforts to develop a diabetes pill are progressing very positively indeed, researchers agree. "If we don't do it, somebody will," says University of Maryland researcher Alessio Fasano, M.D. "The future of people with diabetes will be one without needles."

Implantable Insulin Pumps

For anyone already using an insulin pump worn on the hip, the idea of implanting such a device inside the body might seem hard to imagine, but it's being done—and very successfully, with most patients reporting even better glucose control than that achieved by more conventional means. The implantable pumps are much smaller than the portable devices—only about the size of a silver dollar, in fact—and approximately 800 of them have been implanted since 1980 in a procedure that takes only 30 to 90 minutes and in some cases requires only local anesthesia.

> *The future of people with diabetes will be one without needles.*
>
> —ALESSIO FASANO, M.D.

Pumps generally provide 3 to 4 years of service before having to be replaced, and they can usually go 1 to 3 months between refills depending on the insulin dosages the patient requires. The pumps are expensive, however, costing between $10,000 and $15,000, with another $2,000 to $5,000 for surgery, and while available in Europe, they still are awaiting approval for use in the United States.

MINIMIZING THE DAMAGE

Of course high blood sugar isn't the only problem associated with diabetes. Complications quite literally can extend from head to toe, but rest assured progress is being made against these, too.

Preserving the Nerves

Nerve damage, a debilitating and painful consequence of diabetes, could be a thing of the past if research into *recombinant human nerve growth factor* lives up to current expectations. The substance is a naturally occurring human protein that preliminary studies suggest can restore function to damaged nerves by bolstering their resistance to injury while also enhancing their own mechanisms of repair. Research presently is underway at more than 90 medical centers around the country, including the Albert Einstein College of Medicine in New York.

Protecting the Eyes

There's certainly eye-opening news here as laser therapies are now available that some studies suggest could reduce the risks of blindness caused by diabetes by as much as 60 percent. Scientists also are making progress against eye damage caused by diabetes thanks to their discovery of a substance called *vascular endothelial growth factor* (VEGF) thought to be responsible for the abnormal growth of damaged blood vessels that leads to retinopathy and blindness in the first place. This same substance, paradoxically, is also under investigation as an agent for reestablishing blood flow in diabetics to areas of the body deprived of adequate circulation because of arterial blockage.

> *L aser therapies are now available that could reduce the risks of blindness caused by diabetes by as much as 60 percent.*

Controlling Kidney Damage

In addition to making progress in perfecting the immunosupressant drugs needed to prevent organ rejection, scientists have made the fortuitous discovery that a drug currently used to treat high blood pressure, called Captoprol, can reduce risk of kidney failure in people with type 1 diabetes by as much as 50 percent.

Guarding Against Gastroparesis

Gastroparesis is the decidedly unappetizing condition in which diabetes damages the nerves that control the muscles of the gastrointestinal tract, the result being bloating, loss of appetite, and sometimes nausea and vomiting as food gets stranded in the stomach. Currently the condition is treated with only marginal success with metoclopramide (Reglan) and erythromycin (Propulsid), but in recent studies with mice, the condition was substantially improved when the

animals were given the popular drug for male impotence—Viagra.
According to Christopher Ferris, M.D., of Vanderbilt University, who
helped conduct the study, Viagra appears to work by helping the pyloric valve leading from the stomach to the small intestine relax in much the same way it helps certain key muscles in the penis to relax, thus allowing it to fill with blood. Studies will need to be done with humans before the drug can be recommended for treating gastroparesis, Dr. Ferris says, but it appears to warrant optimism nonetheless.

> *Gastroparesis was substantially improved when the animals were given the popular drug for male impotence—Viagra.*

Preserving Vital Tissue

The letters *AGE* stand for "advanced glycosylation end products," and scientists feel they may be responsible for many of the most serious complications that diabetes can cause. In a chemical process similar to what happens when a piece of meat is browned in a skillet, AGEs develop as molecules of protein in the body combine to form irreversible bonds called *cross-links*. As these bonds accumulate, they can begin to cause blood vessels and other vital tissue in the body to become stiff and eventually dysfunctional, contributing to complications such as retinopathy, nerve damage, skin ulcers, high blood pressure, tissue damage leading to amputations, and even heart attacks and strokes.

Already shown to inhibit the formation of AGEs in animals, a group of drugs called *AGE inhibitors* currently are being tested in more than 100 medical centers to see to what degree they might also be able to prevent or at least delay the progression of certain diabetes complications in humans. Scientists, meanwhile, are working on a new generation of AGE inhibitors they hope will be able to break up cross-links that already have been established. Based on one such drug (ALT-946) that's been able to eliminate cross-links in animals by 80 percent, they remain very hopeful.

Aiding Weight Loss

Yet another area of diabetes research showing promise is the search for drugs to help people with type 2 diabetes control the weight gain so commonly associated with the disease. Weight gain not only can contribute to the onset of type 2 diabetes, it can also result from the disease as the body's impaired ability to use insulin causes excess amounts of this fat-storing hormone to accumulate in the blood. Even when just modest amounts of excess fat are lost, however, major improvements occur. Insulin insensitivity declines, resulting in reduced needs for medication, and blood pressure and levels of bad LDL cholesterol generally come down as well. These are potentially lifesaving benefits, which is why doctors are so fervent in encouraging their type 2 patients to lose weight. It's also one of the reasons why no fewer than 45 of the world's largest drug companies are burning the midnight oil right now to develop medications capable of making weight loss a less daunting task. Diet and exercise should be the mainstays of a long-term weight control program whenever possible, of course, but for certain patients, a little help from a pharmaceutical friend can sometimes be useful.

Several prescription medications are available already—Xenical, for example, which works by inhibiting the absorption of dietary fat, and appetite suppressants such as Meridia, Phentermine, and Bontril—but scientists have better things in mind. They're exploring a naturally occurring hormone called *leptin*, for example, which preliminary research shows may aid weight loss by controlling the appetite center of the brain as it also revs up the body's metabolism. One study with humans found that people given a daily injection of a synthetic leptin derivative (while also slightly restricting their caloric intake) lost 4 pounds in a month, while people on the same diet given a placebo lost just 1 pound. Scientists also are looking into compounds called *beta-3 antagonists* that they're hoping can be made to work like "exercise in a pill" by causing the body to burn more calories even at rest.

So yes, the search for safe and effective medications to aid weight-loss is indeed a fervent one, and understandably so. Obesity is a significant risk factor not just for type 2 diabetes, but for more than 14 other medical conditions including heart disease, strokes, arthritis, liver disease, pancreatitis, low back pain, digestive disorders and urinary incontinence. It also is responsible for an estimated 300,000 deaths every year, so an effective weight loss medication could be a lifesaver in the truest sense of the word.

> *A naturally occurring hormone called leptin may aid weight loss by controlling the appetite center of the brain as it also revs up the body's metabolism.*

Nutritional Medicines

In addition to new drugs, new surgical techniques, and new technologies, expect to also see new food products that will seek to treat diabetes from a nutritional standpoint. One such product, called Level Best, currently is undergoing testing in 20 people with type 2 diabetes under the auspices of the Joslin Diabetes Center of the Harvard University School of Medicine. The product is a beverage and tablet combination to be taken twice daily, with dinner and lunch, that consists of pysllium, ginseng, fructose, barley, chromium picolinate, red yeast rice, and willow bark—all of which have been shown individually to help control blood sugar or blood fat levels in some way.

"Five years ago this science did not exist," says Stacey Bell, D.Sc., R.D., chief scientist at Functional Foods, Inc., makers of the nutritional tonic. "But today, research is telling us that nutrition can help people with diabetes maintain healthy blood sugar and cholesterol levels." The results of the 16-week study being done by the Joslin Diabetes Center should help us know to what degree this is true.

BEST HOPES FOR A CURE

But of course it's a cure for diabetes we all want most, and it's a dream that *will* come true. Scientist aren't confident in saying exactly when yet, but speculative estimates are in the range of 5 to 10 years—right around the corner considering all the centuries the disease has been with us.

Pancreas Transplants: Promising Despite Problems

What would seem to be the most logical solution to curing type 1 diabetes—namely, replacing the organ whose failure is the cause of the disease—is not a new idea: More than 4,000 pancreas transplants have been performed successfully since 1966, most of them in conjunction with kidney transplants, and when they work they can work very well, says Paul Robertson, M.D., director of the Diabetes Center at the University of Minnesota, where about 75 of the surgeries are performed every year.

The problem is that they do not always work. Over half fail, in fact, as the body tries to reject what it correctly perceives to be a foreign object. Even when transplants do succeed, moreover, the side effects of medications patients must take to prevent organ rejection sometimes are as undesirable as diabetes itself—nausea, fatigue, high blood pressure, acne, ulcers, and even damage to the very organ (the kidneys) that the new pancreas otherwise would protect. Because these medications work by suppressing the immune system, moreover, they can increase risks for bacterial and viral infections and possibly even cancer.

Yet another problem is the limited degree to which pancreas transplants can reduce risks of long-term complications from diabetes. While damage to the nerves, eyes, muscles, and kidneys seems to level off several years after transplantation, the symptoms of cardiovascular disease often progress undaunted, possibly because the immunosupressant drugs required to prevent organ rejection also tend to raise cholesterol and triglycerides, researchers say. Then, too, there's the problem of supply being far short of demand: An estimated 1 million Americans with type 1 diabetes are potential candidates for pancreas transplants, but only 1,000 to 1,500 adult organs become available each year.

All things considered, pancreatic transplants show huge potential, but they still have some drawbacks to be worked out before they can be considered a good choice for most type 1 patients. Most researchers agree that unless diabetes is uncontrolled and totally disrupting a patient's life, and unless the transplant includes a kidney transplant as well, undergoing a pancreas transplant simply for the sake of escaping insulin injections or dietary restrictions probably is not worth the risks involved. This may change, however, as new, less harmful ways of preventing organ rejection are found, so there's certainly reason for hope.

> *Islet cell transplants constitute the biggest step toward a cure for diabetes in the past 10 years.*
>
> —HUGH AUCHINCLOSS, M.D.

Islet Cell Transplants: Getting Closer Every Day

Given the difficulties of transplanting an entire pancreas, might transplanting just the insulin-producing beta cells themselves, which occur in small clusters called *islets*, be a better idea? Some very encouraging experiments done at the University of Alberta in Edmonton, Canada, have scientists thinking yes. According to the director of the Juvenile Diabetes Research Fund Center for Islet Cell Transplantation at Harvard Medical School, Hugh Auchincloss, M.D., "Islet cell transplants constitute the biggest step toward a cure for diabetes in the past 10 years." As of June 2000, eight type 1 patients receiving such transplants had been able to forgo insulin for 14 months, and studies of other type 1 patients currently are in progress (discussed shortly).

Instrumental to the success of islet cell transplants has been the use of immunosupressant drugs less toxic than those used with full organ transplants, yet progress in this area still needs to be made, Dr. Auchincloss says. "We don't think it's wise to replace insulin with immunosupressant drugs, especially in children," he notes.

To get around this problem, researchers have been experimenting with ways to encapsulate islet cells in a coating—one that protects the cells from the body's immune system while still allowing glucose to enter and insulin to get out. Some tests of this system have been suc-cessful in animals, but studies with humans have met with difficulties, as the body has shown a tendency to add yet another coating to the encapsulated cells in a process known as *fibrosis*. Scientists remain very encouraged by their progress with micorencapsulation, however, and also another process that improves islet cell survival by accompanying the transplants with stem cells derived from bone marrow.

The problem of getting the body to accept islet cells is indeed a tricky one, yet one "we will be able to solve," says Jeffrey Bluestone, Ph.D., director of the Diabetes Center at the University of California at San Francisco. In addition to encapsulating islet cells, scientists are working on several other novel ways to "trick" the body into accepting these potentially health-giving newcomers with-out having to use such potentially damaging doses of immunosupressant drugs. One especially promising method employs transplanted bone marrow cells to help persuade the body's immune system to be more tolerant of islet transplants, while another method includes transplanting cells from the lymph nodes of the original donor to help give islet cells a more hospitable home. Many of these methods are more than just laboratory pipe dreams, moreover. They're already undergoing human clinical trials, so help is definitely on the way.

> *In addition to encap-sulating islet cells, scientists are working on several other novel ways to "trick" the body into accepting these potentially health-giving newcomers.*

Solving the Problem of Supply: Could Stem Cells Be the Answer?

While transplanting islet cells no doubt will be perfected, scientists still will need to solve the problem of where to get enough of these precious insulin makers, since the supply available from human cadav-ers will fall far short of demand. The use of islet cells from animals is being explored, but also under investigation is developing islet cells from amazing biological oddities called *stem cells*—cells that have yet to differentiate themselves as to what type of organ or tissue they're going to become. Scientists are working on manipulating the genetic structure of these cells so that they become insulin-producing islet cells suitable for transplantation—so suitable, in fact, that they will not arouse the defenses of the body's immune system, thus eliminating the need for immunosuppressant drugs.

Stem cells occur in a variety of organs and tissue in the adult body, but the most workable type, called *embryonic stem cells*, are derived from human embryos that result from test-tube fertilizations. The future of this method of stem cell procreation will depend on the resolution of ethical issues associated with the procedure, but scientists remain encouraged that much will be learned by experimentation with this methodology, nonetheless.

Recently scientists have been successful in deriving especially "coachable" stem cells from bone marrow, for example, and another procedure that grows insulin-producing cells from cells known as precursor cells taken from the ducts of the pancreas itself has raised hopes for an eventual cure even more. "The whole field is exploding," says Bernhard Hering, M.D., associate director of the Diabetes Institute of Immunology and Transplantation and codirector of the Juvenile Diabetes Research Foundation Center for Islet Transplantation at the University of Minnesota. Speaking of the work with precursor cells specifically, "The prevailing view for decades has been that this was not possible, but there's been a major shift in thinking thanks to a number of important contributions recently from key scientific areas." Teamwork. Just as in athletics, it's the key to success in science, as well, Dr. Hering says.

Technology's Answer: The Artificial Pancreas

As promising as the search for a biological cure for diabetes has been, however, it may be a mechanical solution that is achieved first—a continuous and noninvasive (and possibly even implantable) glucose-monitoring system used in conjunction with an implantable insulin pump to effectively mimic how the body controls its blood sugar naturally. When the glucose-monitoring system would sense blood sugar is high, it would signal to the insulin pump to release an appropriate amount of insulin accordingly, and a stable blood sugar level would be maintained based on an ongoing communication between the two.

How far off might such a system be? Not very. An implantable insulin pump already is available in Europe, as mentioned earlier, and several companies already have developed continuous, noninvasive glucose-monitoring systems that are awaiting FDA approval for patient use. What remains is simply to get the two to work in tandem, and it's a pairing that patients would not be unrealistic to expect to see soon, says Harvard University's Dr. Auchincloss. "If I were a 13-year-old with diabetes right now, I'd have my insulin pump hooked up and be asking when they're going to be giving me the other half—the noninvasive glucose monitoring," Dr. Auchincloss says. The artificial pancreas, in other words, might not be as far-fetched as it seems.

PREVENTION AND EARLY DETECTION

Last but certainly not least, scientists are making headway in learning what it might take to prevent diabetes from developing in the first place. Researchers have had success in preventing type 1 diabetes in animals with injections of compounds, including insulin and the enzyme glutamicacid decarboxylase (GAD), that prevent the immune system from destroying insulin-producing cells. How well these injections might work in humans is not yet known, but human trials currently are in progress to help scientists find out.

Scientists also are making great progress in identifying the genes that cause or predispose people to developing diabetes in the first place. Such knowledge could alert people who are susceptible to be especially careful to eat properly and exercise in order to prevent diabetes from developing. It could make for a very effective one-two punch, indeed, researchers say. When the latest scientific technology begins to join forces with good old-fashioned human elbow grease, that's when diabetes will be in the greatest trouble of all.

Appendix: Resource Information

DIABETES ORGANIZATIONS

American Association of Diabetes Educators
100 West Monroe Street, Suite 400
Chicago, IL 60603
Phone: (312) 424-2426 or
   (800) 338-3633
Web site: www.aadenet.org

American Diabetes Association
1701 North Beauregard Street
Alexandria, VA 22311
Phone: (800) 342-2383
Web site: www.diabetes.org

American Dietetic Association
216 W. Jackson Boulevard
Chicago, IL 60606
Phone: (312) 899-0040 or
   (800) 877-1600
Web site: www.eatright.org

International Diabetes Federation
International Association Center
40 Washington Street
B 1050 Brussels, Belgium
Web site: www.idf.org

International Diabetic Athletes Association
1647 West Bethany Home Road, #B
Phoenix, AZ 85015
Phone: (800) 898-4322
Web site: www.diabetes-exercise.org

Joslin Diabetes Center
One Joslin Place
Boston, MA 02215
Phone: (617) 732-2440
Web site: www.joslin.org

Juvenile Diabetes Foundation International
120 Wall Street
New York, NY 10005
Phone: (212) 785-9500 or
   (800) 533-2873
Web site: www.jdfcure.org

National Diabetes Information Clearinghouse
1 Information Way
Bethesda, MD 20892
Phone: (301) 654-3327 or
   (800) 860-8747
Web site: www.niddk.nih.gov/health
   /diabetes/ndic.htm

DIABETES WEB SITES

The Canadian Diabetes Association
www.diabetes.ca

Children with Diabetes
www.childrenwithdiabetes.com

The Diabetes Monitor
www.diabetesmonitor.com

Juvenile Diabetes Foundation International
www.jdrf.org/kids

Online Diabetes Resources by Rick Mendosa
www.mendosa.com/diabetes.htm

Diabetes Web Sites in Other Languages

German: www.uni-leipzig.de /~diabetes

Italian: www.publinet.it/diabete

Korean: www.diabetes.or.kr

Russian: www.diabet.ru

Spanish: www.saludlatina.com /diabetes

Information on Animals with Diabetes

Yes, Morris and Rover can get diabetes, too, as can many other animals. Sites for cats and dogs are as follows:

Cats: http://felinediabetes.com

Dogs: http://pethealthcare .net/html/body_diabetes_ mellitus_in_dogs.html

COMPANIES THAT MAKE DIABETES PRODUCTS

Glucose Meters

Abbot Laboratories
www.abbott.com

Bayer
www.bayerdiag.com

Home Diagnostics Inc.
www.homediagnosticsinc.com

LifeScan
www.lifescan.com

Roche
www.roche.com

Lancing Devices

Owen Mumford
www.owenmumford.com

Insulin Pumps

Disetronic Holding AG
www.disetronic.com

MiniMed Technologies
www.minimed.com

Insulin

Eli Lilly and Company
www.lilly.com/diabetes

Novo Nordisk
www.novonordisk-us.com

Insulin Syringes

Becton Dickinson and Company
www.bd.com/diabetes

Insulin Jet Injector Devices

Activa Brand Products
www.advantajet.com

Bioject Inc.
www.bioject.com

Medi-Ject Corporation
www.mediject.com

Vitajet Corp
www.vitajet.com

Oral Medications

Aventis
(makers of Amaryl)
www.aventis.com

Bristol-Myers Squibb
(makers of Glucophage)
www.bms.com

Pfizer Inc.
(makers of Glucotrol)
www.pfizer.com

Pharmacia & Upjohn Inc.
(makers of Micronase, Glynase, and Glyset)
www.pnu.com

GlaxoSmithKline
(makers of Avandia)
www.sb.com

COOKBOOKS

American Diabetes Association Diabetes Cookbook by Simon Smith, photographer, and Sally Mansfield, editor (DK Publishing, 2000).

The Art of Cooking for the Diabetic by Mary Abbott Hess (NTC Contemporary, 1997).

The Complete Step-by-Step Diabetic Cookbook edited by Anne C. Chappell (Leisure Arts, 1995).

Cooking with the Diabetic Chef by Chris Smith (American Diabetes Association, 2000).

Diabetes Cookbook for Dummies by Alan L. Rubin, M.D., Fran Stach, and Denise C. Sharf (IDG Books Worldwide, 2000).

The Diabetes Snack, Munch, Nibble and Nosh Book by Ruth Glick (American Diabetes Association, 1998).

The Diabetic Dessert Cookbook by Coleen Howard (Avon Books, 1997).

The Good News Eating Plan for Type II Diabetes by Elaine Magee (Wiley, 1997).

Jane Brody's Good Food Gourmet by Jane E. Brody (Bantam, 1992).

The Joslin Diabetes Gourmet Cookbook by Bonnie Polin, Frances Towner Giedt, and the Joslin Nutrition Services Department (Bantam Books, 1994).

Month of Meals: Quick & Easy Menus for People with Diabetes (American Diabetes Association, 1998).

Mr. Food's Quick and Easy Diabetic Cooking by Art Ginsburg (American Diabetes Association, 2001).

101 Nutrition Tips for People with Diabetes by Patti B. Geil, M.S., R.D. (American Diabetes Association, 1999).

The Restaurant Companion: A Guide to Healthier Eating Out by Hope Warshaw and George Blackburn (Surrey Books, 1995).

Tell Me What to Eat If I Have Diabetes by Elaine Magee (Career Press, 1999).

AMERICAN DIABETES ASSOCIATION MEMBERSHIP

Want to become a member of the American Diabetes Association? Not only do you get a monthly issue of their members-only magazine, *Diabetes Forecast* (which includes in-depth articles on topics ranging from recipes to exercise advice to new advances in treatment), you get substantial discounts on all ADA books plus toll-free access to ADA's hot line, set up to answer even your toughest diabetes questions. Dues ($24 annually) go to supporting ADA research in addition to representing the interests of people with diabetes to the U.S. Congress in areas of insurance, research funding, and rights regarding disability and employment. Call (800) 806-7801 for membership information.

Glossary

acarbose An oral diabetes medication that helps control blood sugar levels by inhibiting the breakdown of carbohydrates in the intestine.

ACE inhibitor A drug for lowering blood pressure that is especially useful for people with diabetes who have suffered damage to the kidneys.

advanced glycosylation end products (AGEs) Harmful substances that form when glucose combines with red and white blood cells as well as with other cells and molecules in the bloodstream thus compromising their normal biological function.

alpha cells Cells within the pancreas that make glucagon, a hormone that causes glucose levels to rise.

Amaryl An oral diabetes medication that lowers glucose levels by helping the pancreas increase its output of insulin.

amino acids The molecular building bocks that form proteins.

antibodies Protective substances formed by the body to defend against potentially harmful intruders such as bacteria and viruses.

atherosclerosis A narrowing of the body's arteries due to the buildup of fatty deposits called plaque.

autoimmune disease A condition in which the immune system mistakenly does damage to the body's own organs or tissue.

autonomic neuropathy Damage caused by high blood sugar levels to nerves within organs not under voluntary control, such as the heart, lungs, stomach, and intestines.

Avandia A relatively new type of oral medication for type 2 diabetes that helps lower blood sugar levels by making the body's cells more sensitive to insulin.

beta cells Cells within the pancreas responsible for making insulin.

body mass index A measure of obesity determined by dividing one's weight (in kilograms) by one's height (in meters, squared).

carbohydrates   Chains of sugar molecules prevalent in foods such as fruits, vegetables, and grains that, along with proteins and fats, comprise one of the three basic sources of calories the body uses for energy.

cataract   A clouding of the lens of the eye commonly associated with aging but occurring earlier and more often in people with diabetes kept under poor control.

cholesterol   A form of fat found in foods of animal origin, but also produced by the body. Needed in limited amounts for the production of certain hormones but can lead to narrowing of the arteries if present in large amounts.

Dawn phenomenon   The tendency for blood sugar levels to rise around sunrise due to the release of hormones that reduce the effects of insulin.

Diabetes Control and Complications Trial   The landmark study of type 1 diabetes (but applicable to type 2 patients, as well) that demonstrated that tight control of blood glucose can reduce some of the potential complications of diabetes by more than 70 percent.

ketoacidosis   A condition whereby the body's inability to metabolize glucose forces it to break down fats instead for energy, leading to dangerous levels of acidic by-products called ketones that can cause nausea, vomiting, coma, and even death.

diabetologist   A physician who specializes in treating diabetes.

dialysis   A medical procedure that detoxifies the blood artificially when the kidneys can not properly do the job.

endocrinologist   A physician who specializes in diseases of the glands such as the pancreas, thyroid, and ovaries, and the hormones they produce.

fiber   An indigestible substance found in plant foods that can help lower both blood fats and blood sugar in its soluble form, and assist in alleviating constipation in its insoluble state.

fructose   A type of sugar prevalent in fruits, vegetables, and honey that supplies calories, yet does not cause blood sugar levels to rise as much as table sugar (sucrose), which is half fructose and half glucose.

gastroparesis   A condition involving damage to the nerves of the stomach, resulting in impaired digestion experienced as pain and bloating as the stomach cannot empty as it should.

gestational diabetes   A form of diabetes brought on by pregnancy that usually ends at birth but can increase risks of diabetes in the future.

glucagon   A hormone produced by the alpha cells of the pancreas that has the effect of raising glucose levels in the blood and sometimes is injected to treat cases of severe low blood sugar (hypoglycemia).

glucose   Also called blood sugar, the body's primary source of energy produced mainly by foods containing carbohydrates.

Glucophage   An oral medication used to treat diabetes that works by limiting the amount of glucose produced by the liver.

Glycemic Index (GI)   A measure of the degree to which a food causes levels of glucose to rise in the blood. The higher the number, the greater the food's effect.

glycogen   The form in which glucose is stored by the liver.

Glyset   An oral medication for treating diabetes that works by inhibiting the digestion of carbohydrates.

hemoglobin A1c   A substance in the blood formed when hemoglobin, a protein in red blood cells, combines with glucose, and which can be measured to determine average glucose levels over a period of as long as four months.

high density lipoprotein   Protein particles in the blood that can reduce risks for heart disease by transporting cholesterol from the blood to be broken down by the liver.

hyperglycemia   high blood sugar, usually designated as levels greater than 110mg/dl in a fasting state, or more than 140 mg/dl following a meal.

hyperinsulinemia   A condition of abnormally high levels of insulin in the blood, often characteristic of early stages of type 2 diabetes.

hyperlipidemia   Abnormally high levels of fats (lipids) in the blood.

hyperosmolar syndrome   A condition of extremely high levels of glucose in the blood of people with type 2 diabetes that can lead to coma and death if not treated in time.

hypoglycemia   Levels of extremely low blood sugar, usually less than 60 mg/dl, that can lead to unconsciousness if some form of glucose is not taken.

immunosupression   A suppression of the body's immune system, often activated intentionally by drugs following organ transplants.

impaired glucose tolerance (IGT)   A mild, early form of diabetes (designated by glucose levels between 140 and 200 mg/dl after eating) that frequently leads to a full-blown form of the disease, and which may slowly cause many of the same complications if not brought under control.

insulin   The body's principle hormone, secreted by the beta cells of the pancreas, which allows glucose to enter the body's cells to produce energy. Insulin also allows the body to store excess calories as fat.

insulin reaction   Low blood sugar caused by an excess of injected insulin.

insulin resistance   A decrease in the ability of the body's cells to respond to insulin, and the most common cause of type 2 diabetes.

islet cells   The cells in the pancreas that make insulin.

juvenile diabetes   The name formerly used for type 1 diabetes, the form most common in children.

ketones   The potentially harmful by-products of the body's need to metabolize fat instead of glucose as an alternative source of energy

lancet   A needle used to prick the finger to draw blood for the purpose of measuring glucose.

lente insulin   An intermediate-acting insulin that begins working in 4 to 6 hours and ceases working after 12 hours.

lispro insulin   A very rapid-acting insulin that begins working within 15 minutes of being injected.

low density lipoproteins   Protein particles in the blood that have the unhealthful effect of helping to make cholesterol and triglycerides available for forming deposits on artery walls and hence increasing risks for heart disease.

monosaturated fat   A heart-healthy fat prevalent in olive oil, canola oil, and nuts that does not raise levels of cholesterol in the blood.

nephropathy   Tissue damage within the kidneys.

neuropathy   Damage to nerve cells.

ophthalmologist   A physician who specializes in treating the eyes.

peripheral neuropathy   Damage to nerves within the extremities such as the hands, legs, and feet commonly experienced as tingling, numbness, or pain.

podiatrist   A doctor who specializes in treating problems of the feet.

polyunsaturated fat   A form of fat most prevalent in vegetable oils that does not raise cholesterol levels in the blood but may lower healthful HDLs.

polyuria   Excessive urination.

prandin   An oral diabetes medication that reduces blood sugar levels by stepping up insulin secretion from the pancreas.

proliferative retinopathy   Abnormal development of blood vessels in front of the retina.

saturated fat   A type of fat found in animal foods thought unhealthful for its tendency to raise cholesterol levels in the blood.

sulfonylureas   The first class of drugs to be developed to lower blood sugar by stimulating greater insulin production by the pancreas.

triglycerides   The stored form of fat, which also can circulate in the blood stream and increase risks for heart disease when present in large amounts.

ultralente insulin   A type of insulin that can remain active for as long as 24 to 36 hours.

visceral fat   Fat in the area of the abdomen, thought to be a higher risk for diabetes as well as heart disease than fat located in the area of the hips or thighs.

Index

About the Author

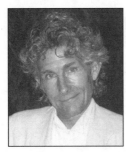

Porter Shimer has been a health and fitness journalist since graduating from Princeton University with a B.A. in English literature in 1971. In addition to 11 books on topics including headaches, back pain, weight loss, herbs, exercise, and depression, he has written a nationally syndicated newspaper column, newsletters and articles for *Prevention, Ladies Home Journal, Mode, Reader's Digest* and *Men's Health*. The father of two daughters—Elizabeth, 25, and Sarah, 20—he lives in Emmaus, Pennsylvania with his wife, Claire, and new son/office mate, Michael, 14 months.

About the Medical Reviewer

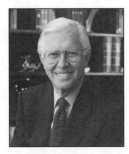

Gerald Bernstein, M.D., F.A.C.P., is an associate clinical professor at the Albert Einstein College of Medicine and a senior endocrinologist at Beth Israel Medical Center in New York. He has served on the national board of directors of the American Diabetes Association, its research foundation, and many national committees. A past president of the American Diabetes Association, Dr. Bernstein is the author of many clinical and scientific papers and the book, *Diabetes: Reducing Your Risk*. He lives with his family in the New York City area.